Physical Medicine and Rehabilitation

GARY A. OKAMOTO, M.D.

Medical Director, Rehabilitation Hospital
of the Pacific, Honolulu, Hawaii and
Head, Division of Physical Medicine and
Rehabilitation, John A. Burns School of Medicine,
University of Hawaii, Honolulu, Hawaii

Formerly, Assistant Professor, Departments of
Rehabilitation Medicine and Pediatrics, University
of Washington School of Medicine,
Seattle, Washington and
Director, Department of Rehabilitation Medicine,
Children's Orthopedic Hospital and Medical Center,
Seattle, Washington

with the assistance of
THEODORE J. PHILLIPS, M.D.

Professor, Department of Family Medicine
Associate Dean for Academic Affairs,
School of Medicine
University of Washington,
Seattle, Washington

1984
W.B. SAUNDERS COMPANY

Philadelphia   London   Toronto   Mexico City
Rio de Janeiro   Sydney   Tokyo

W. B. Saunders Company: West Washington Square
Philadelphia, PA 19105

1 St. Anne's Road
Eastbourne, East Sussex BN21 3UN, England

1 Goldthorne Avenue
Toronto, Ontario M8Z 5T9, Canada

Apartado 26370—Cedro 512
Mexico 4, D.F., Mexico

Rua Coronel Cabrita, 8
Sao Cristovao Caixa Postal 21176
Rio de Janeiro, Brazil

9 Waltham Street
Artarmon, N.S.W. 2064, Australia

Ichibancho, Central Bldg., 22-1 Ichibancho
Chiyoda-Ku, Tokyo 102, Japan

Library of Congress Cataloging in Publication Data

Okamoto, Gary A.

Physical medicine and rehabilitation.
    1. Medicine, Physical. 2. Rehabilitation. I. Phillips,
Theodore J. II. Title. [DNLM: 1. Physical medicine. 2. Rehabilitation. WB 460 041p]

RM700.043 1984   615.8′2   83-19589

ISBN 0-7216-6957-3

Physical Medicine and Rehabilitation   ISBN 0-7216-6957-3

Last digit is the print number: 9 8 7 6 5 4 3 2 1

To Sven-Olof Brattgard, M.D., and his associates of the Department of Handicap Research, University of Gothenburg, Gothenburg, Sweden, who have inspired many people with their leadership, wisdom, and humanitarianism.

CONTRIBUTORS

Editors

GARY A. OKAMOTO, M.D.
Medical Director, Rehabilitation Hospital of the Pacific, and Head, Rehabilitation Medicine Program, Department of Medicine, John A. Burns School of Medicine, University of Hawaii, Honolulu, Hawaii. Formerly Assistant Professor, Departments of Rehabilitation Medicine and Pediatrics, University of Washington; and Director, Department of Rehabilitation Medicine, Children's Orthopedic Hospital and Medical Center, Seattle, Washington.

Assisted by

THEODORE J. PHILLIPS, M.D.
Professor, Department of Family Medicine, and Associate Dean for Academic Affairs, School of Medicine, University of Washington, Seattle, Washington.

Contributing Authors

BRUCE BECKER, M.D.
Director, Rehabilitation Action Center, Sacred Heart Hospital, Eugene, Oregon.

CONSTANCE ARMSTRONG BEYERLIN, M.T.R.S.
Senior Recreation Therapist, Department of Rehabilitation Medicine, Harborview Medical Center, Seattle, Washington.

MARVIN BROOKE, M.D.
Assistant Professor, Department of Rehabilitation Medicine, Emory University; and Associate Chief of Rehabilitation Medicine Services, Emory University Hospital, Atlanta, Georgia.

ROBERT CHESSER, M.D.
Associate Medical Director, Franciscan Rehabilitation Center, Rock Island, Illinois.

JOEL A. DELISA, M.D., M.S.
Associate Professor, Department of Rehabilitation Medicine, University of Washington; and Associate Chief of Staff Education, Seattle VA Hospital, Seattle, Washington.

ALAN J. DRALLE, C.P.O.
Instructor, Department of Rehabilitation Medicine, University of Washington; and Director, Prosthetics and Orthotics Laboratory, University Hospital, Seattle, Washington.

DIANA DUNDORE, M.D.
Clinical Assistant Professor, Department of Rehabilitation Medicine, University of Washington; and Director of Rehabilitation Medicine, Ballard Community Hospital, Seattle, Washington.

JOHN EDWARDS, M.D.
Associate Medical Director, Leon S. Peterson Rehabilitation Unit, Fresno Community Hospital, Fresno, California.

FAY GAYLE, Ph.D.
Director, Parent-Child Learning Clinic, Children's Orthopedic Hospital and Medical Center; and Clinical Instructor, Department of Psychiatry and Behavioral Science, University of Washington, Seattle, Washington.

SHARON GREENBERG, M.O.T., O.T.R.
Instructor, Department of Rehabilitation Medicine, Division of Occupational Therapy, University of Washington, Seattle, Washington.

GLEN A. HALVORSON, M.D.
Physiatry and Sports Medicine, Tucson, Arizona.

DAVID L. HOOKS, Sr., C.R.C.
Director of Vocational Services, Sacred Heart Medical Center, Spokane, Washington.

MARY KEEN, M.D.
Rehabilitation Institute of Chicago, Chicago, Illinois.

RONALD KLEIN, Ph.D.
Clinical Psychologist, Sacred Heart Medical Center, Spokane, Washington.

JAMES W. LITTLE, Ph.D., M.D.
Associate Investigator, Seattle VA Hospital and Department
of Rehabilitation Medicine, University of Washington, Seattle, Washington.

KEITH MacKENZIE, M.D.
Sacred Heart Medical Center, Spokane, Washington.

JOHN F. McLAUGHLIN, M.D.
Associate Professor, Department of Pediatrics, Division of
Congenital Defects, University of Washington; and Chief,
Neuromuscular Clinic, Children's Orthopedic Hospital and
Medical Center, Seattle, Washington.

MARY ANN MIKULIC, R.N., M.S.
Rehabilitation Clinical Specialist, Department of Nursing
and Rehabilitation Medicine, Seattle VA Hospital, Seattle,
Washington.

CHARLES P. MOORE, M.D.
Medical Director, Department of Rehabilitation Medicine,
Salem Hospital—General Unit, Salem, Oregon.

EDWARD O'SHAUGHNESSY, M.D.
Formerly Associate Professor, Department of Rehabilitation
Medicine, University of Washington, Seattle, Washington.

SURINDERJIT SINGH, M.D.
Physiatry Consultant, Tacoma General Hospital, Tacoma,
Washington.

JEFFREY STEGER, Ph.D.
Clinical and Consulting Psychologist, Northwest Medical
Psychological Services, Bellingham, Washington.

TERESA VALOIS, O.T.R.
Chief, Disabled Driver's Program, Occupational Therapy,
University Hospital, and Department of Rehabilitation Med-
icine, University of Washington, Seattle, Washington.

THOMAS WILLIAMSOM-KIRKLAND, M.D.
Department of Rehabilitation Medicine, The Mason Clinic,
Seattle, Washington.

FRANKLIN S. WONG, M.D.
Rehabilitation Action Center, Sacred Heart Hospital, Eugene, Oregon.

KATHY YORKSTON, Ph.D.
Associate Professor, Department of Rehabilitation Medicine, University of Washington; and Chief, Speech Pathology Service, University Hospital, Seattle, Washington.

PREFACE

This manual was developed for physicians in primary care and subspecialties who manage patients with chronic physical disabilities. It is not intended to replace the consultation of physiatrists, orthopedists, and other specialists whose practice routinely involves the treatment of patients with musculoskeletal disabilities. This manual is designed to complement specialty textbooks, references, and journals.

The professional practices of the contributing authors reflect the multidisciplinary nature of the field. Thus, its simple format, practical approach, and action orientation make it a useful resource for nurses, physical therapists, occupational therapists, clinical psychologists, speech pathologists, orthotists, prosthetists, recreational therapists, social workers, vocational counselors, and engineers in rehabilitation.

Residents in training and medical students may use this manual to augment lectures and hands-on experience with disabled patients.

Many of the sections are pertinent to the management of the elderly. Practitioners of gerontology may find useful guidelines in many of the sections.

The overall organization of this manual emphasizes the functional approach to patient management, the concept of independent living, the special procedures and techniques used by practitioners, and the unique features of major musculoskeletal disabilities. The appendices contain frequently needed factual information. Each section suggests guidelines to consider in the management of disabled patients.

GARY A. OKAMOTO

ACKNOWLEDGEMENTS

The editors wish to thank Alice Leighton, Wanda Grande, Pamela White, G. Pat Ford, Carolyn Scott, David Francke, Salvador Betancourt, and Remundo Olivas for their assistance in processing the manuscript. Many thanks are due Justus F. Lehmann, M.D.; Walter C. Stolov, M.D.; Barbara J. deLateur, M.D.; George H. Kraft, M.D.; Eugen M. Halar, M.D.; Wilbert E. Fordyce, Ph.D.; David R. Beukelman, Ph.D.; Diana D. Cardenas, M.D.; and other faculty members of the Department of Rehabilitation Medicine, University of Washington, for their excellence in teaching and research that prepared many of the contributors for the practice of rehabilitation. We must credit the residents in physiatry (1977–1983) for generating the fresh inquiry, enthusiasm, and ideas that gave impetus to this project. We want to acknowledge the cooperation and guidance of Jack Hanley, Al Meier, and John Dyson of the W. B. Saunders Company for their invaluable suggestions and great sense of humor.

Deep appreciation is due Mickey S. Eisenberg, M.D., Consulting Editor, for his kind invitation to participate in the Blue Book Series. His help has been extraordinary.

Special recognition and thanks are due David B. Shurtleff, M.D., and his colleagues of the Division of Congenital Defects, who have taught many of us as an exemplary model for the comprehensive management of children and adults with chronic physical disabilities.

ACKNOWLEDGMENTS

CONTENTS

PART III
TECHNIQUES AND PROCEDURES

PART IV
SPECIFIC CHRONIC PHYSICAL DISABILITIES

FUNCTIONAL PROBLEMS

1

MUSCLE WEAKNESS

Weakness refers to a lack of strength and does not denote a specific cause. For the purpose of this discussion, we shall confine its use to clinical conditions that have resulted from lesions in the cortex, brainstem, spinal cord, anterior horn cell, peripheral nerve, neuromuscular junction, or muscle.

Endurance refers to a person's ability to sustain or continue a task before feeling fatigue. Low endurance may be partly explained by deconditioned muscles, limited cardiovascular performance, poor mental concentration, or adverse effects of medication.

EVALUATION OF WEAKNESS

Even in the presence of obvious physical disability, a careful general and neurologic history should be taken. Inquire about the patient's quality and quantity of ordinary activity at home, work, or school or in the community at large. Ask about walking, sitting, climbing stairs, driving a car, toileting, cooking, or other specific activities. Establish whether "weakness" has improved, stabilized, or deteriorated over two points in time. When appropriate, describe activity in terms of distance, time, or repetitions. Determine those bodily symptoms and signs that precede cessation of the activity, such as pain, shortness of breath, diaphoresis, cramps, fatigue, or frequent rest pauses.

A general and neurologic physical examination should be performed. A musculoskeletal examination is necessary if a physical disability is identified as a possible contributory cause of the patient's weakness. Observe the manner in which the patient walks, stands, sits, lies down, undresses, and enters and leaves the examining room.

Muscle Grading

There are several different systems of grading muscle strength. The "5 to 0" and narrative scales are widely adopted. The physician is encouraged to learn one scale well.

Grade 5 or Normal. The patient can hold or move the body part against gravity and maximal resistance. (It is implied that the body part can voluntarily move through the entire range of joint motion.)

Grade 4 or Good. The patient can hold or move the body part against gravity with minimal to moderate resistance.

Grade 3 or Fair. The patient can hold or move the body part against gravity only. It fails to maintain its position or complete the full range of joint motion against even minimal pressure.

Grade 2 or Poor. The patient can move the body part through the complete range of joint motion with gravity lessened.

Grade 1 or Trace. The patient cannot move the body part at all, although some muscle contraction is visible or palpable.

Grade 0 or Zero. No evidence of muscle contraction is noted on inspection and palpation.

Often, a plus (+) or minus (−) is suffixed to the numerical or term grade in an attempt to describe differences between the major levels of muscle grades.

The physician may proceed to screen muscle function of the upper extremities, lower extremities, back, and neck to determine the extent and nature of the physical disability.

Confounding Factors in Muscle Grading

There are many factors that can lead to false negative or false positive grades in muscle testing. A few are as follows:

A. **Contractured joints.** Restricted joint movement can place a muscle at great biomechanical disadvantage and affect the patient's strength in manual muscle testing or function. For example, knees that lack 25 degrees of full extension will place an inordinate load on the quadriceps during standing and walking. The quadriceps are likely to fatigue rapidly.

B. **Pain.** Always inquire about pain or discomfort during joint movement or muscle contraction. Pain can inhibit maximal contraction and produce spurious weakness in a patient.

C. **Spasticity.** In the presence of uninhibited spinal reflex, muscle grading can be unreliable. For example, manual manipulation of a leg toward extension at the knee may stimulate involuntary knee flexion and create the impression of a strong knee flexor muscle group in a patient with spastic paraplegia.

D. **Hysteria or malingering.** If weakness characterizes a patient with hysteria or one who is malingering, the patient may exhibit little or no effort to show strength. A great show of effort often results in little or no muscle contraction and joint movement. When resistance to flexion or extension is suddenly removed by the examiner, little or no rebound is observed. Manual testing may reveal a wide variety of strength in a pattern inconsistent with the patient's observed ability to carry out functional activities, such as sitting, eating, dressing, or walking.

Comprehensive Evaluation. For a patient with a newly acquired disability or a complex musculoskeletal problem, a comprehensive evaluation may be desirable. As a rule, an occupational therapist has more experience in the assessment of neck, shoulder, elbow, wrist, and hand joints and muscles. A physical therapist is more skilled at the evaluation of trunk, pelvis, hip, knee, and ankle joints and muscles. The therapist may use more quantitative methods of manual muscle testing, such as pulley weights, dynamometers, or isokinetic apparatus (Cybex).

MANAGEMENT PRINCIPLES

A. **Control and coordination.** In conditions of the central nervous system, the patient's perceived weakness is an issue of motor control or coordination or both. The muscle is secondarily affected and thus often deconditioned. The capacity of the muscle to respond to muscle strengthening exercises depends on the specific nature of the physical disability.

For example, in multiple sclerosis, initial therapeutic exercises usually involve repetitive simple or complex movements that do not require great strength. If control or coordination becomes fairly consistent, a trial of muscle strengthening exercises may be considered. A patient with spinal cord injury and paraplegia may respond to strengthening exercises because of a surviving proportion of muscle that is under normal central nervous system control. The loss of normal strength is a result of disrupted neural pathways in the spinal cord that previously allowed for normal excitation and relaxation of the affected muscles.

B. **Orthotics.** Braces, splints, and positional devices may be recommended by a consultant. These orthoses can stabilize a patient's limb and improve its mechanical advantage. For example, a partially weak hand with a flaccid wrist can be braced across the wrist, allowing for fixed extension between 0 and 30 degrees. This can improve the patient's prehension and grasp of objects. Certain types of short leg braces utilize springs to assist the ankle and foot in dorsiflexing during gait, thus avoiding foot drop, toe stubbing, and hazardous falls.

C. **Functional task.** An effective approach toward the rehabilitation of a weak individual is the repeated practice of those functional skills important to the patient, such as walking, climbing stairs, feeding, dressing, or propelling a wheelchair.

Levels of Independence in Therapeutic Exercises

The degree of independence or dependence of a patient carrying out a therapeutic exercise in the clinic or at home may be qualified by any of the following levels of performance:

Passive. There is an absence of any significant active participation by the patient for a given task, function, or activity and full dependence on others (e.g., therapist, spouse, parent, or attendant).

Active Assistive. The patient can actively participate or perform with limitations and requires assistance by a person or device to complete a given task, function, or activity.

Active. The patient independently performs a given task, function, or activity **without** assistance. A patient may perform one task "actively" and require "active assistance" in another task that is more complex or demanding.

Active Resistive. The patient can perform a given task, function, or activity **against** resistance provided by a person or, more commonly, a clinic apparatus (e.g., wall weights, weighted cuffs, dumbbells).

D. **Individual or group muscle strengthening.** Specific strengthening exercises for selected muscles should be done only after the ultimate functional skill or task has been defined and agreed upon as important to the patient. Strengthening exercises "for the sake of something to do" seldom have any real immediate or long-term value for the physically disabled person. Their psychologic importance in the short run should be weighed carefully against potential damage to the patient's adjustment to his or her physical disability.

E. **Fatigue.** Fatigue is the endpoint in most strengthening exercises. Submaximal strengthening, however, may be indicated in some conditions, such as multiple sclerosis in which easy fatigue can be a devastating problem. In muscular dystrophy, overwork or overuse weakness is felt to occur. Strengthening exercises to the point of fatigue may have an opposite effect on the patient's strength or endurance in both of these conditions.

F. **Strength or endurance exercises.** An exercise program of light weights with high repetitions is thought to improve endurance. A program of heavy weights with few repetitions is thought to increase strength. As long as fatigue is attained in each exercise, the clinical outcome may be equivalent. The actual prescription of an exercise program should be properly taught, monitored, and evaluated periodically. Casual or hurried instructions to a patient in a busy office or clinic are unsatisfactory if the physician expects the patient to carry out the exercise program. The patient should understand the indications for continuing or terminating the exercise program. Open-ended programs should be used sparingly.

REFERENCES

Basmajian JV (ed): Therapeutic Exercise, 3rd ed. Baltimore, Williams & Wilkins, 1978.

Cole, TM, Tobis JS: Measurement of musculoskeletal function, Chap 2, pp 19–55. In Kottke FJ, Stillwell GK, Lehmann JF: Krusen's Handbook of Physical Medicine and Rehabilitation, 3rd ed. Philadelphia, Saunders, 1982.

Hoppenfeld S: Physical Examination of the Spine and Extremities. New York, Appleton, Century, Crofts, 1976.

Kendall HO, Kendall FP, Wadsworth GE: Muscles, Testing and Function, 2nd ed. Baltimore, Williams & Wilkins, 1971.

Rosse C, Clawson DK (eds): The Musculoskeletal System in Health and Disease. Hagerstown, Harper & Row, 1980.

Stolov WC: Evaluation of the patient, Chap 1, pp 1–18. In Kottke FJ, Stillwell GK, Lehmann JF: Krusen's Handbook of Physical Medicine and Rehabilitation, 3rd ed. Philadelphia, Saunders, 1982.

2

GAIT DISORDERS

Gait disorders represent any abnormality in bodily movement during walking. There are three categories of gait disorder. The first category involves **upper motor neuron** or **cortical** lesions from, for example, cerebrovascular accidents, head trauma, multiple sclerosis, or spinal cord injury. The second category involves the **primary motor unit.** Diseases of the anterior horn cell, such as poliomyelitis, chronic spinal muscular atrophy, or amyotrophic lateral sclerosis, and the peripheral nerve, such as Charcot-Marie-Tooth atrophy are examples. The third category involves **peripheral musculoskeletal deformities,** such as pain, contractures, discrepant leg length, arthritis, fracture, and dislocated hip.

NORMAL GAIT CYCLE

Normal gait is characterized by smooth, symmetric, effortless movements of arms, trunk, and legs. Cost-efficient shifts in the center of gravity occur naturally. Walking is "automatic" in its development but exceedingly complex in its execution. Walking is highly vulnerable to alterations in the integrity of the neurologic and musculoskeletal systems.

Analysis of Gait. The **stance phase** of gait is characterized by foot contact on the floor and weight bearing. The heel strikes the floor. The midfoot and forefoot soon assume a flat position on the floor. The center of gravity moves over the plantigrade foot. Next, the heel and midfoot leave the floor as hip and knee flexion begin. Push-off occurs as the forefoot leaves the foot.

The **swing phase** of gait is characterized by swinging of the foot through an arc clearing the floor. The phase has begun the moment the forefoot leaves the floor and terminates at heel strike. The pelvis remains level and the hip and knee sweep through flexion and extension (see Fig. 2–1).

EVALUATION OF GAIT ABNORMALITY

A. **History.** Common chief complaints are "My foot drops," "I trip a lot," "My knees buckle," "My shoes wear down quickly." Clarify the problem. Is there pain, swelling, weakness, skin sores, or skin discoloration? Is there a greater or lesser problem in walking over a firm level surface? in walking up or down hills, stairs, or curbs? in getting in or out of cars, the bathtub, or bed?

STANCE PHASE

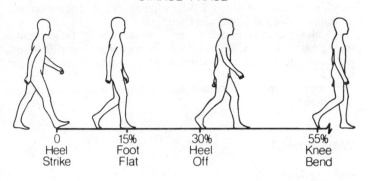

0	15%	30%	55%
Heel	Foot	Heel	Knee
Strike	Flat	Off	Bend

SWING PHASE

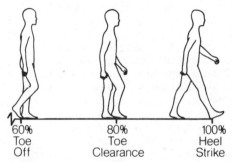

60%	80%	100%
Toe	Toe	Heel
Off	Clearance	Strike

Figure 2–1. The two phases of normal gait are depicted in this illustration. Follow the complete cycle of the right leg.

What has the patient done to improve standing and walking? Review the patient's medical and surgical history.

B. **Physical examination.** Have the patient disrobe for a complete visual inspection of the patient sitting, standing, and walking. For subsequent examination, encourage the patient to wear shorts or swim trunks. Pants, dresses, socks, shoes, and gowns will often hide important physical findings.

Ask the patient to walk up and down a corridor. Except for young children, the examining room is too small. Observe the walking from the front, back, and side. Ask the patient to walk slowly, then briskly, climb stairs, jump, hop, and run. Walking rapidly or uphill often accentuates the gait disturbance.

Compare the affected extremity with the nonaffected extremity. Observe the movements of the head, shoulder, trunk, hips, knees, ankles, and feet. Is the head flexed or rotated? Does a shoulder depress, elevate, protract, or retract? Does the trunk bend, rotate, flex, or hyperextend? Does the pelvis lag, hike, or drop? Does a leg snap at the knee or buckle? Do the feet toe-point, pronate excessively, or stand in varus? Observe the movement at the shoulders, arms, and hands. Do they become rigid, flail, or become tremulous? Are the hands clenched?

Is walking even, symmetric, and narrow in base? Do the shoes show unusual wear? Does the disability appear symmetric? If both sides are affected, does one side appear stronger than the other side?

Perform a careful general, neurologic, and musculoskeletal examination.

MANAGEMENT

Walking Aids

Walking aids are prescribed to improve balance and to provide support during standing or walking. **Canes** provide a minimal amount of support and balance. Up to a quarter of a patient's body weight can be supported by a cane. The cane tip and the patient's two feet create a triangular base of support. For a patient with unilateral lower extremity involvement, the cane is held by the hand of the contralateral side in order to reduce the weight bearing over the affected leg during its stance phase. A pistol-shaped grip on a cane allows for greater comfort, better weight bearing, and more secure handling than the evenly rounded handle of standard canes does. Storage is convenient and inconspicuous. For a greater degree of support or balance, the cane can have three or four points.

Crutches offer greater support, weight bearing, and balance. Forearm crutches (Canadian, Lofstrand) utilize a cuff that encloses the forearm and a handle for the hand to grip. Axillary crutches provide additional support, but may be more unsafe during a fall because of the difficulty the patient will have in tossing the crutch out of the way. Storage is much less convenient for the noncollapsing type than for the telescoping axillary crutches.

Walkers provide the most support and balance. They utilize four broadly spaced posters and are held in front of the patient. A pickup walker requires that the patient have sufficient standing balance and upper extremity strength to coordinate a forward movement by lifting the walker off the floor. A patient with less capability may benefit from a reciprocal hinged or front-wheeled walker, which remains on the floor during gait. A walker can be modified with forearm troughs and handles, which permit weight bearing over the forearm, not the elbow, wrist, or finger joints.

Fitting a patient to axillary crutches is not done casually. The patient's elbow should be held at approximately 30 degrees of flexion. The tip of the crutch should touch the floor 12–20 cm (5–8 in.) to the side of the shoe and in front of the shoe's midpoint.

The height of the axillary crutch should be measured 2.5 cm (1 in.) below the axillary fold. The rubber tip should provide adequate suction and friction. The upright posts and joints should be inspected for breaks and warp.

GAIT TRAINING

Patients with moderate to severe physical disability should be referred to a physical therapist who is trained to teach patients proper techniques in walking and using an aid. There are four major types of gait patterns:

The cane is held on the side with the stronger leg and advanced with the swing phase of the weaker leg. An alternating two-point gait may be prescribed for a patient using two canes or two forearm crutches. The opposite arm and leg move simultaneously. A three-point gait involves the simultaneous placement of the affected leg and the two crutches or canes. Thus, weight bearing on the affected leg is minimized. A four-point alternating gait involves the movement of one cane or crutch initially. The opposite leg then moves and is followed by the movement of the other cane or crutch. The other leg is last to move forward. Three points of support are always present throughout gait.

SPECIFIC GAIT DISORDERS

Spastic Hemiplegia

A quad cane is often prescribed for the patient to hold in the unaffected hand. An ankle-foot orthosis (so-called short leg brace) can be prescribed to protect the ankle, pick up the foot during swing phase, and provide better push-off. Genu recurvatum may also be discouraged during late stance phase. Static stretch exercises for the hip flexors, hamstrings, and gastrocnemius-soleus muscles may be required to prevent loss of joint range due to the underlying spasticity.

Paraplegia

Depending on the severity of the paraplegia, ankle-foot orthoses or knee-ankle-foot orthoses (so-called long leg braces) with appropriate walking aids may be prescribed for both support and balance. Spasticity can make walking difficult and may require extensive treatment. Specific muscle group strengthening exercises and static stretch to preserve joint range of motion may be recommended.

Antalgic Gait

In the case of a painful hip, the cane or crutch is held on the side of the unaffected hip. Stance phase on the painful side will be abbreviated and the center of gravity will be shifted over the affected hip in order to lessen its load. In the case of a painful knee, stance phase will be shortened on the affected side. The cane should be held on the unaffected side but will have relatively less dramatic effect than in the case of hip pain. A patient with a painful midback will walk with small, short steps, rigidity, and guarding. A cane may be helpful.

Lack of Coordination

Athetotic, ataxic, and parkinsonian gait can be improved by the use of walkers. Balance, not support, is often the major problem in safe, independent, functional walking. Repetition, exaggerated steps, audible rhythm, and concentration are important aspects of gait training. Frenkel exercises may be prescribed for a patient with ataxia and emphasize visual compensation for deficits in proprioception through slow, repetitive acts from lying, sitting, or standing position or while ambulating.

Leg Length Discrepancy

A shorter leg may necessitate a shoe lift that will correct 50 to 75% of the height discrepancy. Many people tolerate a difference of 1.8 cm (¾ in.) and elect to go without a lift. For mild to moderate discrepancies, a lift can improve the efficiency and appearance of walking. A large lift can be uncosmetic and heavy. Its use is weighed against its potential benefits in walking.

GAIT ANALYSIS AND MANAGEMENT

Physiatrists, orthopedic surgeons, and physical therapists have the experience and skills to manage patients with complicated disturbances in gait. Today, there are a number of sophisticated motion or gait analysis laboratories equipped and staffed to analyze gait scientifically. Special instruments film or videotape the patient's gait and record the pattern of muscle activity, joint movement, and forces quantitatively. In practice, the vast majority of evaluations involve careful history, physical examination, and trials with walking aids or orthoses in hallways and clinics.

REFERENCES

Blount WD: Don't throw away the cane. J Bone Joint Surg 38(a):695, 1956.
Fischer SD, Gullickson G: Energy cost of ambulation in health and disability, a literature review. Arch Phys Med Rehabil 59:124, 1978.
Hoberman M: Crutch and cane exercises and use, Chap 10. In Basmajian JV (ed): Therapeutic Exercise, 3rd ed. Baltimore, Williams & Wilkins, 1978.

Lehmann JF: Gait analysis, diagnosis and management, Chap 4, pp 56–101. In Kottke FJ, Stillwell GK, Lehmann JF: Krusen's Handbook of Physical Medicine and Rehabilitation, 3rd ed. Philadelphia, Saunders, 1982.

Rosse C, Clawson DK (eds): The Musculoskeletal System in Health and Disease. Hagerstown, Harper & Row, 1980.

Saunders JB, Inman VT, Eberhart HD: The major determinants in normal and pathological gait. J Bone Joint Surg 35(a):543, 1953.

Stolov WC: Normal and pathologic ambulation, Chapter 19. In Rosse C, Clawson DK (eds): The musculoskeletal System in Health and Disease. Hagerstown, Harper & Row, 1980.

3

ORTHOSES FOR THE LOWER EXTREMITIES

An orthosis is an external device for the support, positioning, or protection of a limb, trunk, neck, or any other body part. In common parlance, an orthosis is a brace. There are two major types of lower extremity orthoses. The ankle-foot orthosis (AFO) is the so-called short leg brace. The knee-ankle-foot orthosis (KAFO) is the so-called long leg brace. A person with an amputated limb wears a prosthesis — an artificial limb — not an orthosis.

CLINICAL INDICATIONS

Common indications for the prescription of a lower extremity orthosis are as follows: weak, deformed, spastic, or unstable ankle and/or knee, which less efficiently and effectively functions in walking; and relief from weight bearing at the knee or ankle because of pain, inflammation, or structural instability.

Paraplegia, diplegia, hemiplegia, quadriparesis, and monoplegia may significantly improve by proper bracing. The physician, however, should consider the biomechanical problem of standing and walking before prescribing an orthosis for the patient.

BIOMECHANICAL FUNCTION OF BRACING

Ankle-Foot Orthosis

A. Avoid or minimize toe stubbing as the affected foot and ankle fail to clear the floor during swing phase.

B. Maintain the affected ankle in a neutral position to avoid mediolateral instability and a twisted, sprained ankle.

C. Provide an affected foot with more rigidity in order to improve the patient's ability to push it off the floor during the last part of stance phase.

Knee-Ankle-Foot Orthosis

A. Incorporates the functions of the ankle-foot orthosis and, in addition, stabilizes the knee in the mediolateral direction. If appropriate, flexion of the knee can be prevented by a bail lock or drop lock mechanism and thus provide anterior-posterior stability.

Table 3–1. A COMPARISON OF THE TWO TYPES OF
ANKLE-FOOT ORTHOSES

CHARACTERISTIC	METAL	PLASTIC
Cosmetic appearance	conspicuous	inconspicuous
Sounds or noises	variable	no
Adjustability of ankle angle	yes	no
Interchangeability of shoes	no	yes
Maintenance needs	more	less
Skin tolerance	more	less
Risk of heat rash	lower	higher
Durability, weight, cost	variable	variable
Overall effectiveness and training	comparable	comparable

B. A weight-bearing orthosis is specialized in its biomechanical features and can be prescribed for a patient with a fragile lesion of the lower extremity.

Plastic and metal orthoses are compared in Table 3–1. In either case, the orthosis should not be a stock or "shelf" item. A certified orthotist should be consulted by the prescribing physiatrist or the orthopedic surgeon who has assumed responsibility for the management of the patient's problem in walking.

RELATIVE CONTRAINDICATIONS

1. The use of a walking aid does not assure the patient's safety in standing or walking. Thus, in a patient with poor balance, strength, or coordination, orthosis to the lower extremity may not make any difference and conceivably could aggravate the patient's mobility.

2. Insensate skin particularly over paralyzed limbs makes the patient vulnerable to frank skin breakdown from direct pressure or shear by the orthosis. Skin breakdown can be aggravated by a poor fit, prominent bony surfaces over areas of rough contact, worn-out shoes, heat rash, poor hygiene, fungal dermatitis, a tiny defect in the smooth contour of the orthosis, poor peripheral vascular circulation, and edema.

3. A patient with paraplegia above L2 spinal segment lacks hip flexors and requires a lot more effort to use KAFOs for walking. The goal of walking with KAFOs should be carefully discussed with the patient before embarking on the fabrication of the orthoses and a gait training program. Other rehabilitative goals may take precedence.

4. Anticipated changes at the ankle joint favor the prescription of adjustable metal ankle joints over the fixed ankle angle of plastic AFOs. Conversely, the desire of the patient to use different pairs of shoes favors plastic AFOs, which can be used with two or more

different pairs of shoes of the same heel height. Expense dictates that a patient can afford only one pair of shoes with the fixed metal bracing.

5. A moderately to severely rigid ankle at 5 or more degrees lacking neutral dorsiflexion may not accommodate an AFO without the risk of pain, skin breakdown, and greater instability. A patient with that degree of equinus may require serial casting, motor point blocks, aggressive static stretch, or even surgery before an AFO can be worn.

PRESCRIBING PROCESS

The physician should consult a physiatrist or orthopedic surgeon if it appears that the patient might benefit by bracing. In many cases, a patient with that degree of physical disability is usually being evaluated or followed by a registered physical therapist. If appropriate, the orthosis is prescribed in precise terms. The written prescription is presented to a certified orthotist for fabrication and fitting. Remember that the orthosis is a customized, individualized item.

The prescribing physician should discuss the clinical indications, adverse effects, maintenance, cost, and re-evaluation with the patient and family. The same orthotist who fabricated the orthosis should ideally modify, repair, or renew the patient's orthosis. In most cases, the prescribing physician or physical therapist should check out the orthosis with the patient.

COMMON PROBLEMS WITH ORTHOSES

For **plastic** AFOs, the patient should promptly report to the physician skin intolerance and fracture or buckling of the plastic. In children, growth can make an orthosis obsolete within a year.

For **metal** AFOs, squeaks, loose pins, worn-out springs, missing screws, shoe breaks, broken buckles, and skin intolerance should be reported for remediation.

Musculoskeletal changes can occur from alterations in contractures, ligamentous laxity, pain, spasticity, and strength. Depending on the change, the orthosis may be modified or even discontinued.

The **peroneal nerve** courses around the fibular head and should be avoided by the top trim line or calf band of the AFO. An excessively high AFO can also rub and pressure the popliteal space when the patient flexes the knee in sitting.

Home care of the orthosis may include the following recommendations to the patient: Clean the plastic material with a damp cloth and mild soap, especially over the surface in contact with skin. Lubricate moving metal joints only as directed by the orthotist. Avoid physical abuse of the orthosis, as it is fragile. Take assiduous care of the skin to avoid bacterial or fungal infections. Prevent dependent ankle edema by wearing support hose or elevating the legs at rest. Wear firm, comfortable, solid shoes and use cheaply constructed ones sparingly. Resist do-it-yourself changes in mechanical joints with screws or springs. Do home exercises for muscle strengthening or static stretching as prescribed. Have the use of the orthosis evaluated at periodic intervals.

REFERENCES

Lehmann JF: Biomechanics of ankle-foot orthoses: prescription and design. Arch Phys Med Rehab 60:200, 1979.
Redford JB (ed): Orthotics Etcetera. 2nd ed. Baltimore, Williams & Wilkins, 1980.

4

MOBILIZING THE NONWALKER

Mobility for a disabled person involves movement from one location to another or a change in bodily position in the same location. Walking is not a functional goal for the patient if it cannot be safe, independent, and self-serving. Walking, however, is but one form of mobility.

Mobility can be thought of as a series of progressive movements. **Bed mobility** involves movement of the patient from side to side, prone to supine, supine to prone, supine to sitting, and sitting to supine and shifting in a sitting position. **Transfers** involve movement from bed to wheelchair and back, as well as in and out of chairs, toilet seats, and cars. **Wheelchair locomotion** is the principal means of movement for the patient who does not have safe, independent, functional gait.

CONTRIBUTORY FACTORS OF NONWALKING

A. **Cardiovascular** and **pulmonary conditions**: Chronic obstructive pulmonary disease, coronary artery insufficiency, bronchial asthma, interstitial pulmonary fibrosis, and other diseases.

B. **Obesity**

C. **Visual impairment:** A physically disabled person who has only marginal ability in walking can become nonambulatory if visual acuity cannot be corrected by glasses.

D. **Incoordination:** Parkinson's disease, multiple sclerosis, tumor of posterior fossa, hydantoin intoxication, athetoid cerebral palsy.

E. **High paraplegia:** Patients with a complete spinal cord lesion between L1 and T2 will not have hip flexors and thus will expend enormous energy to walk using KAFOs (so-called long leg braces) and crutches or walkers. Most of these patients eventually rely on mobility devices (e.g., wheelchairs, scooters, carts) as their principal means of locomotion.

F. **Joint deformities in the lower extremities:** Arthritis, contractures, degenerative joint disease, unstable joints of the hips, knees, and ankles.

G. **Kyphoscoliosis:** Severe and progressive spinal deformity in an already compromised person will impair breathing at the same time it creates problems in balance.

H. **Neuromuscular diseases:** Muscular dystrophy, myopathies, myositis; myasthenia gravis, botulism; peripheral motor neuropathies; amyotrophic lateral sclerosis, poliomyelitis, chronic spinal muscular atrophy, and other diseases of the primary motor unit.

I. **Spasticity**
J. **Lower extremity limb deficiencies or amputations**
K. **Immobilization:** For every week of complete bed immobilization, a patient can lose up to 10 to 20% of his or her initial level of muscle strength. By four weeks, 50% of initial strength can be lost. To reverse the process and recondition muscles, however, the rate of return, assuming a patient's maximal effort, is only half as rapid.
L. **Chronic pain**

MOBILITY GOALS

After history and physical examination, the physician should identify the appropriate goals for mobility. Walking should not be regarded as a functional goal if it is likely that it will be unsafe, require 1:1 attendant supervision, and/or occur only in the physical therapy clinic. The adoption of mobility devices, powered or manual, should be seriously considered.

BED MOBILITY AND TRANSFERS

A. **The bed:** A motorized bed with electric button controls allows the patient independent control over the height, head angle, and foot angle of the bed. A firm mattress creates less resistance to rolling or sideways movement and provides a better surface for sitting. A ¼- to ¾-in. plywood plank under a mattress can increase the firmness of an ordinary mattress. Railings can prevent the patient from falling off the bed. The patient can grab the railing in changing position in bed. A change in bed height can also be achieved by blocks under the bed posts or by manual cranks. Overhanging trapeze or slings can provide support by which some patients can pull themselves to a sitting position in preparation for self-care and transfer.

B. **Transfers:** Sitting balance is a prerequisite for safe, comfortable sitting. The specific technique of transfer (e.g., wheelchair or bedside commode) depends on the patient's physical disability. A smooth, hard "sliding" board is sometimes included in the transfer. Standing and pivoting with or without the assistance of another person is the preferred technique in other patients. A physical therapist or occupational therapist is trained to assess and teach patients on the most efficient technique for transfers.

Common transfers involve beds, chairs, sofas, benches, toilets, commode chairs, bathtubs, cars, wheelchairs, and other mobility devices. Depending on the individual case, the therapist may have the patient practice transfers using various seating situations.

Active resistive exercises can help patients in attaining a proficient level of transfers, particularly following prolonged immobilization. Shoulder depressors, adductors, extensors, and elbow extensors can be strengthened.

Standing exercises should be encouraged for the purpose of preparing a patient for standing pivot transfers, provided the patient appears to have the necessary balance, strength, and coordination.

C. **Lifting a patient:** A patient may be severely disabled and require a one- or two-person lift. **Proper lifting techniques** should be taught by a physical therapist, occupational therapist, experienced nurse, or any other trained person to avoid low back injury to the attendant(s). **Mechanical lifts**, such as the Hoyer lift, have a sling in which the patient sits or lies. A hoist and swivel post allow the attendant to lift and lower the patient without risk to the attendant's back. Lifts, however, may be too large for the patient's bedroom or bathroom at home. The straps under the patient and the swinging motion may leave the patient with an uneasy feeling or fear of falling.

D. **Car transfers.** Smaller, fuel-efficient compact cars have created problems for disabled people, who find it difficult to get in and out of them independently. The small doorway and tight cab space make it difficult for the patient to fold and store the wheelchair in the back of the front seat. A medium size two-door sedan is ideal. A **van** with a hydraulic lift is indispensable to a patient who cannot independently propel and transfer out of a manual wheelchair or who uses a powered wheelchair.

E. **The attendant:** Hired attendants, parents, and spouses should be taught proper techniques in transfers. They risk serious low back strain with every transfer. Furthermore, the safety of the patient is always at risk. Osteoporotic bones, fixed deformities, and poor reflexes make many physically disabled patients at great risk for fractures or head injury. Proper equipment, such as adjustable beds, bedside commodes, bathtub benches, wall grab bars, ramps, lifts, and modified lifts, can reduce these risks and improve the efficiency of the transfers.

WHEELCHAIR AS A SEATING AND MOBILITY DEVICE

Conceptually, a wheelchair is a seating device on a platform with wheels. The seating device provides comfortable, safe sitting. The wheels and steering mechanism provide a means of locomotion. However, it is simply not possible for a wheelchair to serve all of the person's household, school, job, recreational, and community activities.

Structural differences among commercially available wheelchairs vary. In weight, for example, a standard wheelchair weighs 21 kg

(46 lb); lightweight, 12.7 kg (28 lb); active duty lightweight, 15.5 kg (34 lb); and heavy duty, 26.8 kg (59 lb). Conventional powered wheelchairs range from a child-sized 45 kg (100 lb) to an adult-sized 90 kg (200 lb). In seat dimensions, the standard adult size measures 45 × 40 cm (18 × 16 in.); narrow adult, 40 × 40 cm (16 × 16 in.); junior, 35 × 32.5 cm (14 × 13 in.).

Because of the growing selection of commercially available mobility devices, a disabled person should be evaluated by a physiatrist, physical therapist, or occupational therapist with the assistance of an equipment specialist. For example, special wheelchairs have been designed for patients with quadriplegia, hemiplegia, paraplegia, and amputations. There are different types of mobility devices for children. Specialized wheelchairs designed for sports, such as basketball, tennis, long distance "running," and sprints, are available. Powered mobility devices can be motorized scooters, carts, or wheelchairs. Most of them are controlled by a joy stick, tiller, or handle bars. More complex control mechanisms are possible for the very severely disabled person.

The **prescription of a mobility device** is an important opportunity for the patient to participate actively. When possible, the patient should be asked to decide on the general type of mobility device, options, modifications, and color.

The **seating component** of the mobility device may involve the following: A firm seat provides a flat level surface for symmetric pelvic weight bearing and even distribution of pressure over the ischial tuberosities; lateral trunk pads prevent the patient from leaning excessively to the right or left; a pelvic stabilizer tucks the pelvis and prevents scissoring; a chest harness minimizes shoulder protraction; head and neck support allows the patient with poor head control to rest the head in an upright, slightly extended manner. Removable desk arms, extended brake levers, and swing-away footrests can be critical in efficient wheelchair transfers.

A patient's capability to locomote in a particular mobility device, manual or powered, **independently,** varies according to the surface, incline, or building. For example, the surface may be grass, mud, gravel, asphalt, linoleum, shag rug, or wood. The incline may be a hill, step, curb, or ramp. The building may include a narrow bathroom, a tight doorway, or a closed door. The general environment may be a home, shopping center, restaurant, basketball court, school, factory, or public restroom.

The prescription should represent a balance or compromise among the following factors: price, funding, delivery time; maintenance, repair; portability, color, durability; accessories; accommodation for expansion or modification.

Funding sources for mobility devices vary. Medicaid, Medicare, and Crippled Children's Services have limited coverage for wheelchairs and other mobility devices. Private insurance policies often limit benefits for a wheelchair to one lifetime purchase. Private foundations like the Muscular Dystrophy Association provide limited benefits for manual and powered wheelchairs. Most benefit plans or programs require some financial participation by the subscriber.

5

LIMB AMPUTATIONS

Every year in the United States, more than 40,000 amputations are performed. Seventy-five to 90% of amputations involve the lower extremities. Over two thirds of patients 50 years or older with amputations suffer from peripheral vascular disease, such as Buerger's disease, arteriosclerosis obliterans, and diabetes mellitus.

Eighty percent of upper extremity amputations are acquired, usually from trauma. In childhood, however, three quarters of affected patients have congenital limb deficiencies or reductions. In contrast to the lower extremities, disease accounts for upper limb loss in only 1 out of 20 cases. Tumors are the cause in nearly half the cases.

DEFINITION

A. **Limb amputation** refers to loss of all or part of an extremity from trauma, disease, or surgery. Thus, by definition, it is acquired.

B. **Limb deficiency or reduction** refers to congenital absence of all or part of an extremity that is evident at birth. It is improper to use the term "congenital amputation."

C. **Prosthesis** is an artificial limb and is best fabricated by a certified prosthetist.

D. **Orthosis** is essentially a brace or splint and is often fabricated by an orthotist. Although some patients with limb deficiencies may utilize orthoses, our discussion will be restricted to prostheses in the management of upper and lower extremities.

UPPER EXTREMITY PROSTHESES

From finger to shoulder, the levels of amputation are transphalangeal, transmetacarpal, transcarpal, wrist disarticulation, long below elbow, short below elbow, very short below elbow, elbow disarticulation, long above elbow, short above elbow, humeral neck, shoulder disarticulation, and forequarter.

In most cases, the orthopedist, general surgeon, or physiatrist works with a prosthetist and occupational therapist in the formulation of the prescription. The patient should understand what a prosthesis can and cannot do for his or her function. In a sensitive fashion, the appearance of the prosthesis is openly discussed and, if possible, the patient is shown a similar artificial limb. Questions of the cost, maintenance, and renewal of the prosthesis should be raised.

A. **Components.** Depending on the level of the amputation, the prosthesis can have a socket, suspension, terminal device, wrist unit, elbow unit, and shoulder unit.

B. **Socket.** It must be customized and developed from a mold of the patient's residual limb. The fit must be total contact in that the socket wall must evenly touch the entire limb skin surface. The socket should be snug. A poor fit can distribute pressure unevenly and create a tourniquet effect. A tight proximal socket can produce edema and discomfort. Acute breakdown or chronic skin irritation can result and become secondarily infected and painful. The socket should be fitted and trimmed until the involved joint is allowed its greatest range of motion.

C. **Suspension system.** In adults, a self-suspending prosthesis is highly desirable and attainable. The socket trim line and shape hangs or purchases the prosthesis on the residual limb. For children and adults with more complex deformities, a strap and harness may be required to suspend the prosthesis. Axillary straps, chest straps, rings, and cuffs may be utilized. The suspension should be comfortable to wear. Ill-fitting straps can produce abrasions and pain and require constant readjustment.

D. **Terminal device.** The end piece of a prosthesis is the terminal device. Crude pinch and grasp can be approximated by a terminal device. The final choice, however, depends on the patient's size, level of amputation, vocation, hobby, and cosmetic appearance. It is not unusual, for example, for a person to own two different terminal devices and interchange them depending on the task at hand. A terminal device can be made of steel or aluminum and its hook lined with neoprene, which is replaceable. Neoprene provides a better grip on objects. The device may measure from 6.9 to 14.7 cm in length and weigh between 54 g (2 oz.) and 368 g (13 oz.). Larger or heavier terminal devices pose special problems for infants, children, and high level amputee adults.

Control of terminal device: How the terminal device is controlled and operated is critical to its use. The selection of the control system is often limited by the nature of the amputation, the patient's ability to learn its use, and the terminal device itself. Voluntary opening terminal devices are widely prescribed and are in a position of pinch unless activated to open up. Voluntary closing devices are also available. Myoelectric controlled hands are prescribed in special situations. Passive terminal devices may be prescribed initially for infants and children.

E. **Wrist unit.** The wrist unit must hold the terminal device securely at variable positions of pronation and supination. Some wrist units allow slight flexion, which can be important in self-feeding, dressing, and undressing. The unit may be oval or circular in shape, vary in size and weight, and quickly disconnect. This last feature may be critical in a situation where the terminal device is dangerously snagged or caught.

Forearm extension. It unites the wrist unit and socket. There are two types. The exoskeletal type is usually made of the same material found in the socket, a polyester resin laminated over layers of nylon stockinette. The endoskeletal type is usually plastic or aluminum tubing with a soft foam and cloth cover. The length of the prosthesis is measured from the lateral epicondyle to the tip of the terminal device. The length should be the same as the distance between the lateral epicondyle and thumb tip on the contralateral sound side. The choice of the forearm extension depends on factors important in the selection of the terminal device.

F. **Systems.** Cables and harness systems are commonly prescribed to control elbow joints or terminal devices. For example, the contralateral sound shoulder isometrically contracts as the ipsilateral shoulder flexes to open the terminal device voluntarily. Electrically powered terminal devices are available and can be quite useful in patients with very short above elbow, shoulder, or bilateral upper extremity deficiencies.

G. **Elbow unit.** An amputation above the elbow will require an elbow joint, which can be locked in variable positions of flexion. An unlocked elbow unit will allow the patient to passively change its angle or to even swing freely. Its control is accomplished by a cable and harness system as described above. Electric elbow units are limited in their use because of weight, cost, and complexity.

H. **Occupational therapist.** The occupational therapist with special experience can work with the prosthetist in teaching the patient to use and care for the prosthesis properly and effectively. Expensive, complicated prostheses unfortunately sit on shelves at home because of inadequate teaching and unrealistic expectations. The therapist may use printed literature, videotapes, or films on use of prostheses to educate the patient.

LOWER EXTREMITY PROSTHETIC MANAGEMENT

The level of amputation can vary from the toe to the proximal hip and be characterized as transphalangeal, transmetatarsal, transtarsal, ankle disarticulation, long below knee, short below knee, knee disarticulation, long above knee, short above knee, hip disarticulation, and hemipelvectomy.

A. **Components.** For the patient with an above or below knee amputation, the component parts of the prosthesis are a socket, suspension, knee joint, and ankle joint.

B. **Socket.** The socket should provide total contact to the residual limb or stump and assume even weight bearing over tolerant areas.

Relief over pressure-sensitive areas, such as the fibular head, distal tibia, distal fibula, and tibial crest, should be carefully fabricated. The socket can be lined with soft padding. However, the hard bare surface of a socket can be tolerated by most patients and allows easy cleaning.

C. **Suspension system.** In the below knee prosthesis, a suprapatellar strap suspends the prosthesis and prevents it from falling off the limb during gait. In some patients, a strap from the prosthesis is attached to a waist belt and is thought to be more for the patient's sense of security than for any real structural suspension.

D. **Foot.** The solid ankle cushion heel (SACH) foot is the most widely prescribed prosthetic foot component. It comes in different sizes. The patient's pair of shoes will determine the exact size of the SACH foot. A different pair of shoes with a different heel height will necessitate a change in the SACH foot.

E. **Above knee prosthesis.** The socket is in total contact with a hard inner surface. In this manner, negative pressure is created between the socket wall and limb. Air leaks from the proximal limb will weaken the suction and its suspension effect. The socket is quadralateral in shape in order to stabilize the prosthesis during different phases of gait. Weight bearing occurs over the ischial tuberosity and gluteal surface, minimizing the impact over the residual limb.

PRINCIPLES OF MANAGEMENT

The primary physician should encourage the patient to be assiduous in his or her care of the prosthesis and residual limb. At visits, the limb should be inspected for signs of chronic irritation, tenderness, infection, acute breakdown, ischemia, muscle strength, joint range, or swelling.

A. **Skin care.** The patient should use fresh, dry cotton or wool socks over the residual limb. The socks should be laundered regularly. Soap and water can be used to clean the socket, which then can be wiped with alcohol or a noncaustic disinfectant. The patient should establish a habit of daily morning and evening inspection of his or her skin. Edema suggests a tourniquet effect. A callus means chronic local pressure and excessive shear. Dark discoloration of the distal limb suggests loss of contact with the socket bottom. Frank skin breakdown and secondary infection can easily occur over the popliteal fossa in the below knee amputee and over the ischial tuberosity or medial groin area in the above knee amputee. In a child, bony growth of a long bone may penetrate the subcutaneous layer and skin of the distal residual limb and require distal excision.

B. **Prosthesis inspection.** The prosthesis should be inspected daily for loose bolts, screws, straps, Velcro, and buckles. The shell may be partly fractured. The prosthesis may be disproportionately heavy, small, or aligned. Shoes may be worn out.

C. **Phantom pain and sensation.** Unusual sensation in the limb is almost universally perceived by patients with acquired amputations. The feeling is perceived as if the total limb were still present. Phantom sensation may dissipate in time or with a full contact socket. Rarely are these sensory experiences a problem for the patient and medications are clearly inappropriate. Phantom pain, on the other hand, can be disabling and is refractory to medication. Only in very rare cases is the phantom pain relieved by excision of a neuroma, revision of a tender scar, or removal of a bony spur. Initial relief is sometimes attained by heat, pressure bandage wraps, and massage. The best treatment, however, is a proper fitting prosthesis with a full contact socket. Again, medications should be avoided because they have no short- or long-term value.

D. **Physical therapist.** A physical therapist with special experience can assist the prosthetist and physician in teaching a patient with a newly acquired limb deficiency proper use and care of the prosthesis. Periodic visits may be requested to trouble-shoot problems related to the patient's use of the prosthesis or to the prosthesis itself.

E. **Energy requirements in walking.** For an adult with a below knee prosthesis, the energy requirement may be a third more than an able-bodied adult. For a patient with an above knee amputation, the same distance may be traversed at a cost of energy two-thirds more than that of a nonhandicapped person.

REFERENCES

Banerjee SN (ed): Rehabilitation Management of Amputees. Baltimore, Williams & Wilkins, 1982.

Bender LF: Prostheses and Rehabilitation After Arm Amputation. Springfield, Charles C Thomas, 1974.

Kostuik JP (ed): Amputation Surgery and Rehabilitation, The Toronto Experience. New York, Churchill Livingstone, 1981.

Setoguchi Y, Rosenfelder R (eds): The Limb Deficient Child. Springfield, Charles C Thomas, 1982.

Sherman RA: Published treatments of phantom limb pain. Am J Phys Med 59:232, 1980.

6

CONTRACTURES

Contractures represent a loss of joint range of motion due to muscle shortening, capsular tightening, or joint incongruity. Burns and other cutaneous or subcutaneous abnormalities may produce contractures. It should be emphasized that muscle tendons are only secondarily involved in contractures and do not shorten. Prolonged immobilization is a common pathway for the development of contractures. Thus, prevention is based on mobilization of the affected joint and maximally conditioned musculature.

CONTRIBUTORY FACTORS IN JOINT IMMOBILIZATION

Spastic or flaccid paralysis of muscles, muscle disease, arthritis, joint trauma, fractures, and agonist-antagonist muscle imbalance can promote prolonged immobilization of joints and eventual contractures. Slings, casts, splints, or braces all potentially can produce contractures.

Chronic or static positioning predispose physically disabled patients to contractures. Sitting in a wheelchair, lying in bed with a pillow under the knees, and walking in a crouched posture, for example, predispose the patient to hip and knee flexion contractures.

PREVENTION

Vary positioning when possible. Encourage prone lying during sleep or use pillows to support paralyzed limbs. Encourage active or passive range of motion at one or more joints no less than twice a day.

A **home program** should be encouraged. Realistically, however, the physician and therapist should be aware of the following factors for optimal compliance: Does the patient appear committed to a home program? Has the patient shown compliance to other medical or rehabilitative recommendations? Is the home situation supportive? Is the program practical, economical, and minimally inconvenient? Does the success of the home program depend on pain tolerance? Can the patient or attendant (e.g., parent, spouse, friend) learn the proper technique? Is there provision for periodic professional monitoring? Are the goals of the home program clearly understood and agreed upon? For example, is the exercise to stretch a muscle group to maintain or increase present joint range of motion?

Resting splints are prescribed mainly to maintain joint range at specific joints, such as the wrist and fingers. Usually, splints are customized for a particular patient and fabricated by an orthotist, occupational therapist, physical therapist, or cast technician. The splint can have plastic, metal, or plaster components. **Braces** or **bivalved plastic casts** can be used to immobilize joints in an attempt to prevent further loss of joint range, particularly at the ankles and knees. Poor skin tolerance or low pain threshold is frequently the reason why splints, braces, or bivalved casts are discontinued by patients.

TREATMENT

A. **Goals.** Develop goals for the treatment of a contracture. How many degrees of joint range do we wish to achieve? What functional value is the improvement of the particular joint range? What is the time frame for treatment? Who will evaluate progress? How often should evaluations occur?

B. **Relative contraindications.** Passive manipulation of joints can result in serious injury to bone or tissue. The prescribing physician and therapist should be aware of osteoporosis, bleeding disorder, heterotopic bone formation, acute arthritis, ligamentous instability, fresh fractures, pain, insensate tissue, and the quality of muscle. (Is it dystrophic, myopathic, inflamed?) Because pain is an important feedback signal to a patient undergoing aggressive stretch to muscle and joint capsule, the clinician should be very attentive in the manipulation of a patient who is unable to communicate, comatose, heavily medicated, or insensate or who is a child.

C. **Static stretch.** Stretch of muscles can be accomplished by steady manual extension or flexion at the affected joint. Special traction devices can be rigged to apply stretch for periods of 30–45 minutes b.i.d.–t.i.d. **Deep heat** may be applied during or immediately after static stretch in order to increase the response to therapy.

D. **Serial plaster casts.** A cylindrical plaster cast can be applied over a limb in order to stretch muscle. It should be changed every 7–14 days. Progress should be measured by a goniometer and, hopefully, show 5 to 10 degrees at every cast change. It may be discontinued because of pain, skin intolerance, or impediment to self-care or locomotion.

E. **Orthoses.** Plastic or metal braces can have mechanical joints or locks that allow changes in the angle (degrees) of relative flexion or extension. An orthotist, occupational therapist, and physical therapist are able to fabricate certain types of orthoses.

F. **Peripheral neurolytic blocks.**

G. **Surgery.** Tendon release, tendon lengthening, tendon transfer, myotomy, capsulotomy, fasciotomy, and osteotomy have been performed in the face of a fixed contracture, which is refractory to conservative methods. **Caution:** The release of an agonist group of muscles can result in the development of a contracture in the previously "silent," "underpowered," antagonist muscle(s). A hip in severe flexion contracture, for example, undergoes complete severance of superficial and deep hip flexors. Spastic, previously overpowered extensors are now unopposed and could produce an extension contracture at the hip, which would create a problem in sitting. The possibility of adverse effects following surgical remediation of contractures should always be considered before surgery.

H. **Maintenance of gains.** Once gains in joint range are made by any or all of the previous procedures, the patient should undergo a home program of maintenance. Such a program often involves lying in a certain position, manual stretch twice a day by a family member, night resting splints, and follow-up by the prescribing physician and therapist. Without such a program, significant gains can be lost within months.

7

SPASTICITY

Spasticity is a symptom complex characterized by hypertonic muscles, hyperactive deep tendon reflexes, clonus, abnormal spinal reflexes, and muscle spasms in flexion or extension. A spastic limb is velocity-dependent in that rapid passive manual manipulation of a joint exaggerates resistance to that movement. Conversely, much slower manipulation meets with less resistance. The loss of normal inhibition over spinal or supraspinal reflexes and hyperexcitable stretch reflexes partly explain spasticity.

Spasticity is commonly observed in patients with upper motor neuron dysfunction, such as spinal cord injury, brain injury, multiple sclerosis, cerebral palsy, and cerebrovascular accident.

Muscle cramps, spasms, fasciculation, rigidity, dystonia, athetosis, and ataxia may be seen in patients with spasticity but do not characterize it per se.

EVALUATION

Establish the presence or absence of spasticity and other disorders of movement. A neurologic and musculoskeletal examination should follow the history and general physical examination.

Determine the influence of spastic symptoms on the patient's function in specific activities at home, work, or school. In mobility, is standing, transfer, walking, or wheelchair use less safe or efficient? In driving a motor vehicle, do leg spasms interfere with the controls? In self-care, are dressing, undressing, grooming, and hygiene made more difficult? In toileting, are intermittent catheterization or bowel programs interrupted? In skin care, do spastic movements predispose bony surfaces to breakdown? Socially, do spasms cause embarrassment or undue attention?

The quantification of spasticity has eluded easy or simple measurement. The degree of spasticity of a patient fluctuates, depending on a myriad of factors, and is at best subjectively evaluated by the clinician. From a rehabilitative standpoint, however, the issue is what specific motor activities are significantly affected by spastic symptoms. Thus, a careful record of various functional activities is important in managing spasticity.

To the unaware evaluator, a spastic individual may be found to have extraordinary strength in the presence of fair to poor coordination of that particular limb. For example, rapid manual testing of elbow flexion can excite flexor stretch reflexes and create the impression of voluntary strength at that joint. **In the presence of spasticity, manual muscle testing may be very unreliable.**

The **serial measurement of joint ranges of motion** is important. Joint range can be insidiously lost. When spasticity cannot be effectively controlled by slow, deliberate movement at a joint, temporary local anesthetic block of the peripheral nerve innervating the specific spastic muscle(s) may be useful.

Stress can aggravate spastic symptoms. Anxiety, fatigue, infection, skin breakdown, obstipation, ill-fitting garments, fractures, and trauma represent a few medical, surgical, and psychologic factors that can aggravate spasticity. On the other hand, relaxation, rest, sleep, and robust health tend to minimize the aversive influence of spasticity.

MANAGEMENT

Correct **aggravating factors.** For example, splint fractures, treat urinary tract infection, remove pressure from a skin sore, relieve a fecal impaction, loosen a tight-fitting elastic band, or encourage restful sleep to avoid daytime fatigue.

Reduce **psychologic or emotional tension.** Teach the patient to deal with tension, fright, and anxiety. Exercises for relaxation or self-hypnosis may be helpful. Some patients need help from a counselor, social worker, psychologist, or psychiatrist with experience and knowledge about the patient's physical disability.

Consultation from a physiatrist, neurologist, or orthopedist may be appropriate in the initial and periodic evaluations of a patient with significant spasticity. An occupational therapist or physical therapist, or both, may be invaluable in working directly with the patient on learning ways to overcome or compensate for the ill effects of spasticity.

Static stretch to joints can minimize the risk of serious muscle and joint capsular contractions. Rapid movement of a limb should be avoided. Excessive manual power can tear muscle and fracture osteoporotic bone. Infrequent, brief, passive stretch is generally worthless. Static stretch at home once or twice a day is minimal exercise for joints at risk for progressive loss of joint range.

Inhibition of spinal or supraspinal reflexes can be accomplished by positioning devices, orthoses, or special manipulation.

Customized orthoses can position joints to discourage spastic movements and to allow functional use of limbs. Less expensive, "off the shelf" orthoses may aggravate spastic symptoms and should be prescribed and checked only by an experienced clinician.

Purposeful, voluntary, selective motor control can be taught to many patients with spasticity. The physician should understand that patients need to relearn motor control and require much practice over a long period of time under qualified supervision and monitoring.

Medication. Currently, there is no miracle drug for the treatment of spasticity. Three widely prescribed antispasmolytic drugs—

dantrolene, diazepam, and baclofen—have had limited success. The physician who is unfamiliar with their individual use should consult a physiatrist or neurologist.

Because patients have spasticity due to a permanent physical disability, the prescription of a drug requires assessment at 2- to 6-month intervals. Pre-drug observations regarding the effect of spasticity on specific functions should be recorded and followed in order to minimize highly intuitive and subjective decisions to stop or continue medication. Side effects or adverse effects may appear and warrant prompt discontinuation. The same clinical effect may be maintained at smaller doses or require a boost in amount. The beneficial effect may diminish with time despite increasing daily doses.

Placebo tablets or capsules may be indicated in some cases to justify continued use of a drug with questionable clinical value.

Dantrolene sodium (Dantrium) inhibits the efflux of calcium released into the sarcoplasmic reticulum triggered by membrane depolarization. Thus, dantrolene targets the muscle, not the neuronal pathways of the peripheral nerve or spinal cord. Adverse effects include nausea, diarrhea, fatigue, weakness, dizziness, and drowsiness. It should be given with caution in patients with severe myocardial disease.

Idiosyncratic or hypersensitivity reactions involving the liver have detracted from the value of dantrolene. Hepatotoxicity appears to occur mostly in women, patients over 35 years, and patients with pre-existing liver disease. Patients on estrogen therapy or taking 400 mg or more of dantrolene daily are also at greater risk. Liver function tests should be ordered prior to dantrolene use to screen for pre-existing hepatic dysfunction. During the period of increasing doses, liver function tests should be obtained biweekly. Subsequent tests should be ordered every 2–4 months. The drug should be discontinued if there is no improvement in 6 weeks.

The usual optimal safe dose ranges between 100 and 400 mg divided into 4 doses daily. Gradual increments of dantrolene should begin at 25 mg P.O. daily and increase over a 2- to 6-week period. Daily doses above 400 mg should be given cautiously and only in responsible patients who can obtain liver function testing conveniently. Doses above 600 mg daily should be discouraged. The drug is available in 25-, 50-, and 100-mg capsules.

Diazepam (Valium) is a benzodiazepine and probably inhibits presynaptic impulses at the spinal cord level, as well as at supraspinal or brainstem sites. Because of its many side effects and potential risk of drug abuse, diazepam should be carefully prescribed. The prescription should never be left open-ended. Adverse effects include sedation, drowsiness, fatigue, ataxia, weakness, light-headedness, and anxiety. It is contraindicated in narrow angle glaucoma and during the first trimester of pregnancy.

Patients on large doses can exhibit withdrawal on abrupt discontinuation. Overdosage results in cardiorespiratory depression.

The usual daily dose is 20–40 mg divided into 2 or 3 doses. The initial dose should start at 2–5 mg P.O. daily, increasing every 2–5 days. Whereas doses as high as 60–80 mg daily have been prescribed, the abusive and addictive nature of diazepam makes such a schedule highly undesirable, except in desperate cases. The drug is available in 2-, 5-, and 10-mg tablets.

Baclofen (Lioresal) acts on the presynaptic mechanisms and probably inhibits the release of excitatory transmitters in the spinal cord. Baclofen is an analog of gamma-aminobutyric acid (GABA). It appears to be more effective in patients with spastic flexor spasms or patterns. Success has been more consistently achieved in patients with spinal cord lesions or multiple sclerosis. Adverse effects include sedation, drowsiness, nausea, weakness, dizziness, confusion, headache, constipation, muscle ache, and ankle edema. Because baclofen is excreted by the kidneys, a depressed renal function should mean relatively lower doses.

Its use in patients under age 12 has not been approved by the Food and Drug Administration. Its effect on pregnancy and breast milk is not known. Baclofen may lower the seizure threshold and should be prescribed with caution in patients with known seizure disorders. Its discontinuation should be gradual in order to avoid hallucinations, disorientation, or irritability.

Overdosage can result in profound hypotonia, cardiorespiratory depression, somnolence, seizures, vomiting, and coma.

The usual adult maintenance dose is 40–80 mg in 4 divided doses. Few patients derive significant benefit from doses as high as 100–160 mg. Begin baclofen at 5 mg b.i.d. with gradual increments every 5–7 days. The drug is available in 10-mg scored tablets.

For each of these drugs, the antispasmolytic effect may influence the patient's musculoskeletal function, particularly if spasms are used to facilitate control of a limb. Abrupt withdrawal may precipitate paradoxical increases in spasticity. The initial adverse symptoms of sedation, dizziness, weakness, or drowsiness usually dissipate with time but may jeopardize safe driving or job-related tasks for a period. Alcohol and drugs affecting concentration and alertness can aggravate these adverse side effects. Baclofen and diazepam do not have the risk of fatal organ toxicity as dantrolene does for the liver. It is not known whether the three drugs have any teratogenic or untoward effect on the developing fetus. Their use should be contraindicated in pregnancy. The safety and effect in children under 12 years are not clearly known.

Peripheral nerve blocks or intramuscular neurolysis (motor point blocks) can selectively decrease spasticity of muscle groups of the upper and lower extremities. For example, a block of the obturator nerve can reduce hip adductor spasticity for up to 3–6 months. Intramuscular neurolysis of the triceps surae can reduce the equinus deformity at the ankle.

Orthopedic or neurosurgical procedures. When conservative, nonsurgical methods fail to control severe spasticity and function might improve considerably with the reduction of spastic symptoms, surgical procedures should be considered.

Previously performed procedures for spasticity management have included the following: Myotomy; release, lengthening, or transfer of muscle tendon; and peripheral neurectomy. Posterior rhizotomy involves interruption of the sensory afferents and anterior rhizotomy, the motor efferents. Bischoff dorsal longitudinal myelotomy from spinal segment L1 to S1 interrupts the afferent-efferent spinal reflex arcs for the lower extremities and relatively spares the reflex arcs for the bladder and bowel. Other types of myelotomies have been performed. Cordectomy is almost never performed for spasticity management.

Continuous neural **electrostimulation** is highly controversial and still under investigation.

However "minor" the procedure appears to be, the primary physician should insist that the surgeon have experience in the management of spasticity. Initial benefits may be neutralized by the appearance of previously "silent" antagonistic muscle groups, recontracturing of the muscle or joint capsule, failure to re-educate the patient in selective motor control, poorly stated functional goals, profound muscle atrophy, loss of bladder and bowel stability, and complications related to the surgery itself.

REFERENCES

Merritt JL: Management of spasticity in spinal cord injury. Mayo Clin Proc 56:614, 1981.

Stolov WC: The concepts of normal muscle tone, hypotonia, and hypertonia. Arch Phys Med Rehabil 47:156, 1966.

Young RR, Delwaide PJ: Spasticity, Parts I and II. New Engl J Med 304:28, 96, 1981.

8

PRESSURE SORES

Pressure sores (decubitus, bed sore, pressure ulcers) are localized areas of tissue necrosis produced by ischemia from excessive external pressure and blockage of capillary blood flow. Pressure sores usually occur over bony prominences. Seldom, however, is direct pressure alone the cause of skin breakdown. Distortion and shear of the skin are two other major mechanisms of tissue trauma in patients with a "pressure" sore.

PATHOGENESIS

Pallor is the initial response of tissue to local ischemia. When pressure is relieved, signs of **erythema, edema,** and punctate **hemorrhages** often are seen. The overlying skin may slough and evolve into a well-circumscribed area of necrosis within 3–5 days. Bacterial **infection** exacerbates the process and can eventually reach exposed fascia and bone. **Sepsis** and **death** can occur.

The distribution of pressure through the tissue below the external source is cone-shaped, with its apex near the surface. The break in the skin can deceptively appear as a superficial wound that, in fact, may be deep and cavitating.

Grading pressure sores. Grade I is superficial redness and induration, which persist 24 hours or more after the cessation of pressure. **Grade II** involves blisters or very superficial breaks in the skin. Erythema and induration persist. **Grade III** involves the dermis. **Grade IV** is breakdown of overlying skin, subcutaneous layer, fascia, and muscle. Bone is spared. **Grade V** involves frank osteomyelitis.

The **pelvic** area and **lower extremities** account for nearly 9 out of 10 pressure ulcers. Ischial tuberosities, vertebral spinous processes, sacrum, coccyx, trochanters, knees, heels, dorsum of the foot, toes, and malleoli are frequently the sites for pressure sores. The occiput, scapular spine, and elbows are other areas of high risk.

Predisposing factors include paralysis and insensate skin; poorly perfused tissue due to edema, vascular disease, or irradiation; limited tissue healing due to anemia, negative nitrogen balance, weight loss, decreased vitamins or minerals, or dehydration; fecal and urinary soiling, poor skin hygiene, and perineal dermatitis; and altered mental status, such as confusion, depression, stupor, and coma. Creases, rigid seams, snaps, buckles, straps, and shoes can be a source of pressure and account for unusual superficial configurations in the skin.

INITIAL EVALUATION

Establish that the skin lesion is secondary to direct pressure. Consider shear, friction, burns, impetigo, contact dermatitis, and even self-inflicted wounds, all of which require different treatment.

Grade the pressure ulcer. Identify contributory factors. In general, assuming that treatment is optimal, a Grade I pressure ulcer takes 3–5 days to heal; Grade II, 10–14 days; Grade III, 3–8 weeks; Grades IV and V, 3–6 months. It is not unusual for an experienced physician or nurse to take 1–2 weeks to determine the exact limits of a serious pressure sore. Superficial necrotic tissue requires vigorous debridement for proper evaluation.

Plain radiographs of underlying bone are important in pressure sores that are chronic, recurrent, or severe in nature. **Radiographic sinogram** should be done on suspected Grade IV and V pressure ulcers to rule out tracts to joint capsules and bursa and to define the limits of the lesion. **Bone scans** may be considered but can be falsely positive for osteomyelitis in the presence of inflamed adjacent soft tissue. If the initial technetium bone scan is negative, a gallium scan may be ordered next. If surgery is required to expedite healing and control infection, a **bone biopsy** may be important in establishing the diagnosis and causative bacteria.

After 1–2 weeks of stabilization, surgical debridement and exploration may be important in directing treatment in the severe cases.

Gram stains, cultures, and antibiotic sensitivities in vitro should be obtained initially, particularly if the wound appears infected. In a hospital setting, cultures are ordered every 1–4 weeks. Blood cultures are obtained only if sepsis is suspected.

MANAGEMENT

Keep pressure off the involved area. For a pelvic ulcer, consider a 10-cm thick layer of foam cushions lying over the bed. The blocks of cushions, however, are split or separated by 10–40 cm of space directly under the area of skin breakdown. For a sacral, coccygeal, or ischial pressure sore, the patient may require turning every 2–6 hours in prone or side-lying positions. For ischial sores, the patient should avoid sitting or flexed supine lying. For ankle, foot, or toe pressure sores, foam boots held by Velcro straps or a wide, thick foam "bracelet" proximal to the ankle can reduce pressure considerably. For the elbow lesion in a patient who must assume a prone position, a plaster case with a cutout over the elbow wound may allow the patient to support the chest off the mattress during activities.

A patient with multiple or serious skin breakdown should be evaluated by an experienced nurse or physician. Inappropriate positioning, inadequate turning schedules, ineffective techniques in pressure relief, and poor control over aggravating factors can cause further deterioration of the wound.

Remove necrotic debris frequently. Clip loose debris with tweezers and iris scissors. Make up a 1:1 solution of hydrogen peroxide and water. Apply the solution generously with cotton swabs or clean gauze pads. Allow for effervescence. Repeat the process if necessary. Rinse with copious amounts of normal saline. Hydrogen peroxide is caustic to healthy tissue.

Apply **wet-to-dry dressings** every 4–12 hours. Moisten a square gauze pad with normal saline and apply it directly over the pressure ulcer. Lay a dry gauze pad over the damp one. As the wet gauze dries, the necrotic debris becomes entrapped and adheres to it. If bleeding occurs with the removal of the dried gauze pads, soak them with normal saline prior to removal. Use a stockinette, tube gauze, or Montgomery straps to hold the gauze dressings in place. Frequent changes in adhesive tape can result in contact dermatitis. Discontinue wet-to-dry dressings when necrotic debris and drainage are no longer major problems in wound care.

Consider **hydrotherapy.** Treat large craters with hydrotherapy 1 or 2 times daily. Water Pik (Teledyne) is portable and appears to debride effectively by pulsating jets of water. The device can be used at home and requires little teaching. Whirlpool and Hubbard tanks allow for deep immersion of the affected region of the body. They require assiduous maintenance and are utilized exclusively in hospitals. Some patients have been successfully managed at home, using bathtubs with Jacuzzi-type devices.

Enzymes, such as Elase (Parke Davis), Travenase (Flint), and Collagenase (Armour) have been used to hasten the separation of exudates and devitalized fibrinous tissues. These enzymes spare the protein of viable cells and, theoretically, avoid injury to healthy tissues. Treatment should be limited to 1 or 2 applications daily over a 7- to 14-day period.

When exudate is profuse, hydrophilic beads of dextranomer (Debrisan, Pharmacia) can be applied to the wound 1–4 times daily. The beads are rinsed or irrigated off before sprinkling fresh beads.

Eschar should not be unroofed as a rule. If little subcutaneous tissue underlies the eschar, aggressive mechanical removal of the eschar may unnecessarily expose uninfected bone or fascia and inadvertently remove contiguous healthy epithelium. If signs of abscess or cellulitis implicate the eschar, excision of it is promptly warranted. Healthy tissue will form beneath a dry, noninfected, protected eschar, which will eventually slough off. Its loose edges can be clipped with scissors and forceps.

Surgical excision in the operating room may be indicated in large, devitalized, infected pressure ulcers. The procedure can be staged and involves simple debridement, full excision, bony removal, or cutaneous muscle flaps. A plastic surgeon should be consulted. Surgery does **not prevent** the recurrence of pressure ulcers. Surgery does expedite wound healing. The surgical scar, however, is not normal healthy skin and is more prone to skin breakdown.

Whether the patient is in hospital or at home, a visual inspection of the wound should take place 2–4 times a day. A goose neck hand-held mirror should be available to the patient for personal use.

When healthy granulation and epithelial tissue have appeared, discontinue the wet-to-dry dressing and begin nonadherent dressing on a b.i.d. schedule. Pigskin has been used to facilitate healing. Because its effectiveness varies it should not be routinely used. A clear, semipermeable adhesive film (Op Cite, TJ Smith & Nephew Co.) can be applied over a delicately epithelialized wound to reduce the need for frequent dressing changes. Exudate and gross infection are relative contraindications for Op Cite use. Moisturize the new skin with nonallergenic lotions b.i.d. Avoid desiccated skin.

After the best of efforts, the healed-over wound may be extremely fragile, parchment thin, and chronically irritated by the slightest shear, pressure, or distortion.

Precaution. A table lamp with an incandescent bulb has been utilized to dry weeping, draining wounds. Improperly positioned and unprotected bulbs have accounted for many inadvertent burns of insensate skin. It should **not** be routinely recommended for home treatment or inadequately supervised hospital use.

PREVENTION

The hallmark of pressure ulcer management is **prevention.** The patient and family should be taught the principles of skin care and wound prevention. The **earliest reliable sign** of excessive pressure is an area of reddening that persists for 20 or more minutes after the cessation of pressure, such as sitting. The patient should be encouraged to establish the health habit of visual inspection of body parts at risk for skin breakdown at least twice a day. A goose neck hand-held mirror should be routinely prescribed to most patients with paraplegia or quadriplegia.

For the paraplegic or quadriplegic individual, it is usually necessary to perform **wheelchair pressure releases** every 20–30 minutes. An inconspicuous timer or wrist watch with a buzzer is recommended for the patient who responds to auditory cues.

A proper **cushion** for the wheelchair can be critical in the prevention of ischial or sacral decubiti. A 7.5-in. latex foam cushion with a 2.5-cm cutout over the sensitive region may be initially prescribed. High-density foam cushions or foam sandwiches may be recommended as well. Other types of cushions are composed of rubberized air cells (Roho) or gel.

To provide a level, flat, firm surface for symmetric weight bearing over the ischial tuberosities, a thin plywood piece or insert should be considered. The naughahyde or heavy plastic seats used in most wheelchairs become bowed with use and predispose the patient to pelvic obliquity in sitting. A physiatrist, physical therapist, or nurse specialist may be consulted before the final prescription for a cushion is written.

The **bed** or **mattress** can be important in relieving pressure over areas of the body irritated during sitting or standing. Synthetic sheepskin, egg crate liner, alternating pressure pad, water-filled flotation pad, and foam blocks can be effective. A water bed may be prescribed for some patients.

The decision to hospitalize a patient with a pressure ulcer depends on a number of factors. Sepsis, Grade III–V ulcers, lack of home attendant services, multiple aggravating problems, severe underlying physical disability, history of noncompliance, or suspected self-mutilation favor admission. A supportive home environment and compliant patient, however, can defer or obviate hospitalization in the majority of cases of skin breakdown.

There is no substitute for a regimen based on removing the precipitating cause, correcting aggravating factors, rigorous debridement of necrotic tissue, control of infection, and judicious but sparing use of surgery, time, and preventive measures. Claims of rapid cure with a single topical medication, for example, are rarely justified.

REFERENCES

Galpin JE, et al: Sepsis associated with decubitus ulcers. Am J Med 61:346, 1976.
Kosiak M: Etiology of decubitus ulcers. Arch Phys Med Rehabil 42:19, 1961.
Morgan JE: Topical therapy of pressure ulcers. Surg Gynecol Obstet 141:945, 1975.
Shea JD: Pressure sores, classification and management. Clin Orthop 112:89, 1975.

9

URINARY TRACT INFECTION AND NEUROGENIC BLADDERS

A neurogenic bladder is at risk for infection due to an impairment in host defense mechanisms against bacterial invasion. The risk of clinically significant infection is influenced by the adequacy of host defenses, the size of inoculum, and the virulence of the organism.

Host defense mechanism. The higher osmolarity and the lower pH of urine have greater antibacterial activity than urine with lower osmolarity and high pH. Phagocytes in the bladder mucosal lining may entrap bacteria. The size of the bacterial inoculum may be effectively reduced by a bladder that completely empties with voiding and has continuous flow of sterile urine.

Impairment of host defenses. Residual urine of more than 20% of the bladder volume before voiding increases the risk of bacterial colonization. An infected kidney will intermittently or continually seed the bladder urine with bacteria.

Vesicoureteral reflux involving residual or stagnant infected urine will lead to recurrent or chronic infection of the renal parenchyma. **Calculi** will form the nidus for urinary tract infection in either the bladder or the kidney. Bladder calculi are often associated with a foreign body (e.g., an indwelling Foley catheter) and infection by a urea-splitting organism (e.g., *Proteus mirabilis*), producing an alkaline urinary pH. Staghorn calculus and other renal stones are frequently associated with *Proteus, Staphylococcus*, or *Pseudomonas* infections. The calculi are generally composed of magnesium and ammonium phosphate.

Urethral or **suprapubic indwelling catheter** can act as a potent nidus for infection and calculi formation. The urine is usually colonized with bacteria.

Bacteriuria. The unresolved issue is whether or not "asymptomatic" bacterial colonization of bladder urine warrants antibiotic treatment. Many patients with neurogenic bladders have utilized indwelling catheters for years and have demonstrated persistent asymptomatic bacteriuria. Bacteriuria of renal origin is invariably associated with systemic evidence of tissue invasion, particularly in the presence of vesicoureteral reflux.

EVALUATION

Urinalysis and **urine culture with sensitivities** should be obtained in a workup of fever in a patient with a neurogenic bladder. Sterile technique is recommended. A straight in-and-out catheterization or a suprapubic needle tap can be performed. If the patient has an indwelling catheter, it should be removed and a specimen of urine obtained as a fresh, new catheter is inserted through the urethra. These tests should be obtained at least annually and more frequently, as the clinical situation dictates.

In the presence of an ileal diversion, ileal cutaneous ureterostomy, or vesicostomy, a **double lumen catheter technique** should be used to obtain a urine specimen. A #18 French straight catheter and a #8–10 French feeding tube can be used. The larger outer catheter is inserted initially under aseptic conditions and preparation. Next, the smaller inner catheter is threaded through the larger catheter in order to obtain a specimen of urine.

Antibody-coated bacteria may fluoresce and suggest renal tissue infection. Some evidence, however, suggests that prostatic infecting bacteria also fluoresce. Bacteria that are negative for fluorescent staining may be considered noninvasive.

Bladder washout (Fairley test). Catheterize the bladder through the urethra and obtain urine for urinalysis and urine culture. Lavage the bladder with 2 L of saline. Obtain a urine specimen for culture every 10 minutes postlavage for a 30-minute period, or three specimens. A primary bladder infection usually results in negative or negligible colonies on each of the three specimens. A primary upper tract infection is substantiated by postlavage colony counts that approach or approximate prelavage culture results.

Radiologic methods of evaluation begin with a supine film of the abdomen (the so-called K.U.B.), which can show radiopaque calculi of the kidneys or bladder. **Ultrasonography** can also pick up stones. **Intravenous pyelogram** (IVP) can detect structural defects, including hydronephrosis, pyelectasis, hydroureter, bladder or calyceal diverticula, or calculi. The degree of architectural distortion of the renal calyceal system can suggest the relative acuteness or chronicity of the infection. Obstructed or delayed flow of urine can best be evaluated by IVP. **Renal tomography** can be combined with IVP to enhance its sensitivity. Serious allergenic reactions to the iodine salt in the IVP contrast medium do occur.

A **cystogram** can define the bladder contour well and detect vesicoureteral reflux. Retrograde filling of various ureteral or vesical diversions can be accomplished with contrast medium and catheterization. In the presence of infected urine and reflux, the procedure can lead to acute pyelonephritis and possibly sepsis. Asymptomatic infections of greater than 100,000 colonies should be treated first **before** the cystogram or loopogram is performed.

Cystoscopy can be helpful in visualizing stones and bladder diverticula that might have eluded radiologic or ultrasonographic evaluation. **Ureteral catheterization** (Stamey procedure) can differentiate lower from upper tract infection and right from left kidney-ureter infection.

MANAGEMENT

Prophylactic medication. In the presence of an indwelling catheter, there is little evidence to prove that any medication taken daily will actually prevent bacteriuria. Urologists, physiatrists, and infectious disease specialists vary in their use of medication to "suppress" bacterial colonization in the asymptomatic patient with an indwelling catheter. Methenamine mandelate, methenamine hippurate, and ascorbic acid have been recommended.

Methenamine mandelate (Mandelamine) is a combination of mandelic acid and methenamine, which can produce a urine pH of 5.5 or less. At this pH, methenamine is hydrolized to ammonia and formaldehyde, the active antibacteriocidal agent. Because of the tendency of the urine to remain at higher pH levels, methenamine mandelate is less effective against urea-splitting organisms, such as *Proteus* and *Pseudomonas aeruginosa*. The drug is reputed to be effective against gram-positive and gram-negative organisms. When the outflow of urine is rapid, the drug is less effective. Renal failure is a major contraindication. Occasional nausea occurs in some patients. The usual dose is 1 g P.O. q.i.d., or 4 g total daily. It is available in 0.25-, 0.5-, and 1.0-g tablets and suspensions of 250 or 500 mg/5ml.

Methenamine hippurate (Hiprex) can acidify urine and allow the methenamine ingredient to undergo hydrolysis to ammonia and formaldehyde. Renal or hepatic failure is a contraindication to its use. Nausea and skin rash have been reported. The dosage is 1 g P.O. b.i.d. It enoys the distinct advantage of fewer tablets per daily dose. It is available in 1-g scored tablets.

Ascorbic acid (vitamin C) is taken to keep urine at a pH of 5 or less. There is evidence to suggest that at the recommended dosage, ascorbic acid cannot reliably and consistently maintain an acid pH in urine, leucocytic phagocytosis may be impaired, and calculi formation may be facilitated. Loose stools to diarrhea occasionally occurs. The dose schedule is 0.5 g P.O. b.i.d. to 1 g P.O. q.i.d.

Methenamine mandelate and ascorbic acid have been used in combination at recommended dosages. Theoretically, ascorbic acid prepares the urine by acidification and thereby facilitates the hydrolysis of methenamine into formaldehyde.

Daily bladder lavages can reduce the risk of calculus formation in the bladder. The acid solutions, however, are regarded as an irritant to the bladder mucosa and as a possible factor in the development of thickened vesical walls. **Suby's G solution** consists of citric acid monohydrate 32.5 g; magnesium oxide anhydros 3.84 g; sodium carbonate 4.37 g; dissolved in 1 L of water at pH 4.

Renacidin 10%: mix citric acid 156–171 g, D-gluconic acid 21–30 g, magnesium acid citrate 9–15 g, purified magnesium hydroxycarbonate 75–87 g, calcium carbonate 2–6 g, and water 17–21 g, producing a 300-g bottle.

Urologic G solution consists of citric acid hydrous U.S.P., sodium carbonate anhydrous 430 mg, magnesium oxide 380 mg, pH 4, in every 100 ml.

A 30-ml bolus of solution can be lavaged b.i.d. or Q12 hours. Urologists and physiatrists vary in their individual opinion of the preventive potential of daily acid lavages in patients with indwelling catheters.

Symptomatic infection. Acute systemic episodes of urinary tract infection or pyelonephritis involve bacterial invasion of tissue. Fever, chills, anorexia, nausea, vomiting, and dark, foul smelling urine can characterize a symptomatic infection. In patients with spinal cord injury above T4–6, autonomic dysreflexia may appear. Painful micturition and low abdominal cramps may occur in patients with partly or completely normal sensory feedback from the bladder and urethra. Urinalysis reveals pyuria, bacteriuria, and, occasionally, hematuria. Colony count of a single organism usually exceeds 100,000 in the significant infection.

Because patients with neurogenic bladders often experience recurrent urinary tract infection, the employment of antibiotics should be done judiciously and, whenever possible, only after the antibiotic sensitivities are known. Treatment length varies from 3 to 14 days, depending on the prescribing physician's policy.

Intermittent catheterization. When performed properly at home, work, or school, the sterile or clean technique of intermittent catheterization should entail a low risk for bacteriuria. When **persistent bacteriuria** is diagnosed, the physician should consider inadequate technique, dirty or worn out catheters, unsanitary storage of fresh catheters, and abnormalities of the urinary tract, such as vesicoureteral reflux, calculi, prostatitis, diverticuli, and hydronephrosis. Experts differ in the management of persistent asymptomatic bacteriuria in a patient on intermittent catheterization. Short-term antibiotic treatment or chronic urinary acidification has been recommended when colony counts exceed 100,000 with or without symptoms.

Acute, episodic, symptomatic infection should always be treated with the appropriate antibiotics. Because of lowered host resistance and the physical vulnerability of patients with neurogenic bladder, an acute infection may lead to hospitalization for antibiotics and hydration by intravenous route. Frequent emptying of the bladder is also critical in reducing the risk of vesicoureteral reflux and urinary stagnation.

10

URINARY INCONTINENCE AND NEUROGENIC BLADDER

A **neurogenic bladder** results from a disruption of the afferent or efferent pathway, or both, connecting the bladder to the controlling centers of the spinal cord, brainstem, and cortex.

CLASSIFICATION

Uninhibited bladder allows for normal filling. The patient perceives bladder fullness and voiding. However, the person cannot inhibit the detrusor contraction, making voiding imperative. Residual urine may or may not be present. The uninhibited bladder is seen in patients with cerebrovascular accident, brain tumor, head injury, multiple sclerosis, parkinsonism, and enuresis.

Reflexic bladder contracts reflexively and is often accompanied by a small volume capacity. Relatively high residual urine volumes may occur. The reflex arc is at the spinal cord level. The patient voids involuntarily. The reflexic bladder is associated with spinal cord trauma, inflammation, tumors, and multiple sclerosis.

Detrusor-external urethral sphincter dyssynergia. Normally, the external urethral sphincter relaxes when the detrusor muscle contracts. In dyssynergia, the inhibition of the external urethral sphincter is incomplete or absent. The bladder empties incompletely or not at all. Dyssynergia is usually observed in reflexic bladders. Patients usually have traumatic spinal cord injury or multiple sclerosis.

Areflexic bladder fails to contract in the face of increasing bladder volumes. There are three types. Dysfunction of the upper motor neuron can temporarily result in an areflexic bladder, which eventually evolves into a reflexic-type bladder, seen in early spinal cord injury. Disruption of the central reflex arc can produce absent bladder sensation, negligible intravesical pressure and, frequently, flaccidity of external urethral and anal sphincters. This situation is seen in spinal cord tumors or trauma and multiple sclerosis. Lesions of the afferent loop can produce a large-capacity bladder with absent detrusor contraction. The person may initiate voiding voluntarily. Retroperitoneal surgery and peripheral neuropathy (e.g., diabetes mellitus, lues, and other causes) can be associated with this kind of areflexic bladder.

ANATOMY

The **fundus** of the bladder is a major part of the **detrusor**, a three-layered smooth muscle that forms the internal sphincter.

Parasympathetic end organs are scattered throughout the bladder with a greater concentration in the fundus and are terminations of the pelvic nerve (n. erigentes). These end organs are under acetylcholine control, and their preganglionic neurons reside in the S2–4 spinal cord segments.

Alpha and **beta sympathetic** end organs are scattered about the fundus and vesical neck. The beta receptors are more prominent in the fundus and are antagonists to the parasympathetic end organs. The alpha-adrenergic receptors are more prominent in the trigonal proximal urethral area. They are terminals of the hypogastric postganglionic outflow from T12 to L2.

Trigone and bladder neck. The trigone forms the base of the bladder. When the bladder contracts, the detrusor opens the internal sphincter and bladder neck. Ureteral orifices pierce the trigone at the extremes of its base, and the internal sphincter orifice constitutes the trigonal apex. Parasympathetic end organs in the bladder neck are of minimal clinical significance. A major concentration of postganglionic alpha receptors is situated in the area. The neural transmitter is norepinephrine. The action of these sympathetic end organ receptors is contraction of the vesical neck and proximal urethra.

Innervation of the bladder-urethra and external sphincter (micturition neural axis) can be characterized by the following: The micturition control is situated in a specific area of the motor cortex. **Loop I**, the cortical-pontine-mesencephalic loop, primarily inhibits the detrusor and can function at the subconscious level.

Loop II, the pontine-mesencephalic-sacral nuclei loop, primarily controls the duration of detrusor contraction. These afferent and efferent columns run in the area of the reticulospinal tract. Uninhibited, inefficient voiding pattern can occur.

Loop III, the pelvic–pudendal nuclei loop, primarily inhibits or excites the end organs. Stimuli from cephalic centers are integrated through the somatic and autonomic nervous systems. Detrusor–external sphincter synergy is a Loop III activity. At the instant of micturition, the external sphincter relaxes as the detrusor contracts. Sudden increase in pressure (e.g., coughing) will excite the contractile sphincter activity more. Lack of this reciprocal relationship is known as dyssynergy. In addition, as the bladder fills, the detrusor is stretched and generates afferent stimuli. Reflexively, the efferent stimuli contract the detrusor for voiding.

Loop IV, motor cortex–pudendal nuclei loop, primarily controls the external sphincter. The medial motor cortex can directly inhibit or excite external sphincter activity voluntarily.

Diseases or lesions involving any portion of the micturition neural axis can result in a neurogenic bladder.

Functional impairment can consist of the following: an inability to void voluntarily, to recognize the voiding urge, to completely empty the bladder, or to interrupt involuntary voiding. Sudden increase in intra-abdominal pressure (laughing, coughing, Valsalva's maneuver) can trigger incontinence. Voiding may be felt imperatively or urgently. Involuntary voiding is usually characteristic of a neurogenic bladder.

EVALUATION

Mechanical alterations of the distal urinary tract can produce abnormalities in micturition in patients with neurogenic bladders. A discussion of prostatic hypertrophy, urethral stricture, bladder neck relaxation, external urethral sphincter injury, and other mechanical lesions is outside the scope of this section but should be considered in evaluating the neurogenic bladder.

The intensity of urologic evaluation should be individualized. Costly urodynamic assessments do not replace careful clinical observation and basic urologic screening. Although physicians may learn to perform cystometrography and other urologic tests, the interpretation of data is critical in proper management. Consultation should be sought.

Efficiency of micturition. Determine the amount of urine retained in the bladder following a void. After the patient voids, catheterize the bladder immediately. If it is feasible, observe urination in terms of initiation, flow, stream, volume, and termination.

Radiologic evaluation. The **excretory urogram** or **intravenous pyelogram** is sensitive in detecting abnormalities in renal and ureteral morphology. **Renal tomograms** can clarify renal structure and function more sharply when used with excretory urograms. When the IVP is unsatisfactory or the patient is allergic to the contrast medium, a **renal scan** may be considered next. **Retrograde urethrocystograms** can reveal vesicoureteral reflux and, in some cases, a qualitative estimation of voiding efficiency. Static evaluation involves catheterizing the bladder and filling it with contrast fluid by gravity. A radiograph is taken when filling has ended. Another x-ray film is taken 10 minutes later. If possible, voiding and postvoiding x-ray films should be obtained. Dynamic evaluation involves cinefluoroscopy or a videotape urogram in which the movement of contrast medium can be visualized as the bladder contracts following its instillation by catheter. Activity of the bladder, ureters, and vesical neck can be observed. Subtle ureteral reflux can be detected.

Cystometrography is the standard and basic physiologic study for bladder function. It records the changes in intravesical pressure in response to filling. Pressure is measured in cubic centimeters (cm³) of water pressure. Water cystometrograms involve instillation of sterile saline through an indwelling catheter by gravity flow. Classically, the intravesical pressure was monitored by the column of water in a manometer connected to the Foley catheter via a Y-connector. Currently, pressures are measured by a transducer and simultaneously recorded on graph paper. Carbon dioxide cystometrograms can be similarly done but are thought to be less physiologic than the use of sterile saline. Cystometrography has been useful in the classification of bladders.

Urodynamic evaluation is the physiologic study of micturition and can include the following: cystometrography, urine flow rate, external urethral sphincter electromyography, bulbocavernosus reflex electromyography, voiding urethral pressure, and provocation tests by changes in temperature or position. The urodynamic study is useful in a patient with a mixed, changing, or complex dysfunction, which is often seen in patients with incomplete spinal cord injury, myelomeningocele, or multiple sclerosis.

External urethral sphincter. An electromyographic needle can be inserted through the skin of the perineum just lateral to the prostatic apex in the male or through the mucosa of the vestibule just lateral to the urethral orifice in the female. An indirect measurement can be obtained by anal plug or needle electrode activity, which presumably reflects the same pudendal nerve influence manifested by the external urethral sphincter.

Bulbocavernosus reflex. The presence of the reflex implies an intact afferent and efferent neural pathway of the sacral spinal segments 2, 3, and 4. The reflex can be elicited in 70 to 80% of normal, able-bodied people. The dorsal nerve of the penis can be cutaneously electrostimulated. An electrode in the ischiocavernosus muscle will pick up activity. During cystometrography, the physician can tug on the retention catheter. Afferent pathways will carry the stimuli from the bladder neck and urethral area to the conus medullaris of the spinal cord. Synaptic efferent pathways will excite the external urethral and anal sphincters, producing electromyographic activity.

Urethral pressure is another way of measuring external sphincter activity. Pressure readings can be obtained at any site between the bladder neck and the urethral meatus. A dynamic comparison of pressure gradients can be made between the intravesical and urethral pressures, particularly at the site of the external sphincter.

Temperature provocation test (iced cystogram) is a selective test that can be useful in differentiating bladder neck (internal sphincter) obstruction from external urethral sphincter dyssynergia. Iced radiopaque contrast is instilled into the bladder through a catheter. A positive test results if the bladder neck opens and the contrast fluid is expelled. A negative test means that the bladder neck is closed and the contrast fluid retained in the bladder.

Positional provocation test. A cystometrogram performed in the traditional supine position may provide spurious information. The detrusor may behave differently when the patient assumes a standing or sitting position. A cystometrogram with the patient lying, sitting, and standing should be done, particularly in incomplete lesions of the spinal cord and in demyelinating diseases.

MANAGEMENT

The **goals** of bladder management are to establish a relatively safe pattern of urine storage and evacuation and to attain socially acceptable urinary continence.

Uninhibited Bladder, Efficient-Type

This bladder is relatively efficient in that urine residual is usually less than 20% of the normal bladder capacity. If the detrusor response is delayed by an anticholinergic drug during urodynamic testing, consider the following:

1. **Chloropheniramine maleate** 8 mg and **phenylpropanolamine hydrochloride** 50 mg (Ornade) 1 spansule P.O. Q12 hours. Side effects are drowsiness and dryness of the mucous membrane of the nose, throat, and mouth. Severe hypertension or coronary artery disease contraindicates its use.

2. **Propantheline bromide** (Pro-Banthine) is available in both 7.5- and 15-mg tablets. Up to 45–90 mg P.O. divided into 3 or 4 daily doses can be taken. Side effects are decreased perspiration, mydriasis, constipation, thirst, and dryness of the mouth, nose, and throat. Glaucoma, obstructive intestinal disease, and myasthenia gravis are contraindications.

3. **Oxybutynin chloride** (Ditropan) combines anticholinergic effects and direct antispasmodic activity in smooth muscles. Dosage is usually 5 mg P.O. b.i.d.-q.i.d. Side effects are pupillary dilatation, dryness of mouth, and constipation. Contraindications are glaucoma, obstructive intestinal disease, and myasthenia gravis. It is available in 5-mg tablets or 5 mg/5 ml syrup.

4. **Imipramine hydrochloride** (Tofranil) is not an anticholinergic but has enjoyed success in the management of uninhibited bladders due to cerebral lesions. The reflexive bladder of spinal cord injury can sometimes be helped. The site of action is unclear. It is a tricyclic antidepressant and has improved nocturnal enuresis in able-bodied children. It may increase urethral resting pressure by stimulating alpha-adrenergic receptors. Imipramine is available in 10-, 25-, and 50-mg tablets. The total dosage is 75–200 mg P.O. daily divided into 3 or 4 doses. Side effects are mouth dryness, mydriasis, restlessness, insomnia, and bone marrow depression. Concomitant use of monoamine oxidase inhibitors are contraindicated.

Uninhibited Bladder, Inefficient-Type

This uninhibited bladder is inefficient in that postvoid residual urine is often 20% or more of normal bladder capacity. If the detrusor response is altered by an anticholinergic drug, consider the following:

1. Imipramine hydrochloride: If postvoid residual urine increases, discontinue imipramine and consider the second alternative.

2. Intermittent catheterization. An anticholinergic (e.g., propantheline bromide) is often necessary to produce urinary retention. Intermittent assisted or self-catheterization can then be instituted every 4–6 hours.

Reflexive Bladder

This bladder is typically associated with patients with spinal cord injury.

1. **External collecting device** and leg bag should be considered as the management of choice in a male patient with an efficient reflexive bladder.

2. An **indwelling catheter** may be tried after an external collecting device and intermittent catheterization have failed. A Silastic urethral indwelling catheter is preferred. Anticipate bacteriuria. In females, the urethra is likely to dilate gradually and result in leakage around the catheter due to positional changes or detrusor contraction. Increasing the size of the catheter is ultimately self-defeating. Consider anticholinergic drugs to ablate the detrusor response. A consulting urologist may suggest periurethral injection of Teflon to provide resistance to further dilatation. In the male, submucosal false passages, urethritis, prostatitis, and epididymitis can account for significant morbidity.

3. **Intermittent Catheterization Program (ICP)** involves bladder catheterization at timed intervals, allowing for storage and evacuation of urine and simulating normal voiding. Catheterization may be performed independently or with the assistance of a spouse, parent, or attendant. The frequency of catheterization is dependent on the rate of bladder filling. Bladder volumes of 300–350 ml should be emptied. The average patient will require a Q4–6 hour schedule of intermittent catheterization. The risk of bacterial infection and urethral trauma is important to minimize with sound technique.

There are two techniques, a hospital-based and a home-based intermittent catheterization. The hospital-based technique is sterile. A gowned, masked, and gloved attendant is usually needed. Sterile disposable catheter kits are used with a #14 French straight catheter. The genitalia are cleansed and a sterile area isolated for catheter insertion, using a sterile forceps.

The home-based program involves **clean intermittent catheterization (CIC).** The person should wash the hands, cleanse the urethral meatus with povidone-iodine (Betadine), and hold the catheter with one hand 3 in. from the tip. The catheter should be slowly inserted until urine flows. After the bladder is completely emptied, the catheter should be slowly removed.

The acidity or alkalinity of the urine should be checked daily with a pH tape purchased at any drugstore. The pH should ideally be maintained between 5 and 6. If the pH is 7 or more, a urinary tract infection or dehydration should be suspected.

Intermittent catheterization and anticholinergic medication should be considered in the female who has problems with frequent or continuous dampness. Allergic dermal reactions to the iodine-containing solutions warrant a change to other cleansing preparations.

Detrusor–External Sphincter Dyssynergia

1. **Anal stretch:** The patient stretches the anal sphincter in order to inhibit the external urethral sphincter. This maneuver, however, may also inhibit the detrusor. The feasibility of this method may be demonstrated at the time of diagnostic urodynamic assessment. A Credé maneuver should accompany the anal stretch to overcome any detrusor inhibition.

2. Intermittent catheterization with or without anticholinergic medication.

3. **External sphincterotomy** is often recommended when the dyssynergia leads to high intravesical pressure in excess of 40 cm H_2O. The transurethral surgical interruption of the external sphincter will ablate the obstructing intraurethral pressure and allow reflex micturition in response to detrusor contraction. The patient will then have been rendered incontinent and will require an external collecting device. A small percentage of male patients (1–3%) will become impotent following external sphincterotomy.

Areflexic Bladder

1. **Bethanechol** (Urocholine) is the drug of choice in stimulating detrusor activity. The dose should be gradually increased to an oral dose of 25–60 mg q.i.d. The dose may be gradually decreased until postvoid residual urine volumes are less than 100 ml. The drug is available in 5-, 10-, 25-, and 50-mg tablets. Abdominal discomfort, salivation, flushing of the skin, and a "hot" feeling are side effects. Bethanechol is contraindicated in hyperthyroidism, pregnancy, peptic ulcer, asthma, epilepsy, and parkinsonism.

2. **Credé** and **Valsalva** maneuvers should stimulate a truly denervated bladder to contract. Timed voidings may be taught to the patient. By the clock, the patient can empty the bladder and minimize embarrassing episodes of unexpected urinary incontinence associated with sudden increases in intra-abdominal pressure.

Decompensated Bladder

This bladder is refractory to medication, timed voiding, externally applied bladder pressure, and intermittent catheterization. In this case, the major goal is the attainment of a low pressure conduit for urinary excretion.

1. **Indwelling catheter,** #14–16 French **Silastic** type, can be attached to a leg bag or a night bag. This simple method has been successfully and safely employed by many patients over many years. Anticipate bacteriuria, stone formation, and vesicoureteral reflux. Monitor the patient closely. In female patients, anticipate dilatation of the urethra and urinary leakage around the catheter.

2. **Suprapubic catheter** may be permanently inserted through a cystostomy, which is surgically created in the midline just above the pubis. **Silastic** catheters should be used (Foley retention, Pezzer, Malecot suprapubic catheters). The distal tips spread or balloon out, providing sufficient resistance to prevent the catheter from falling out of the stoma and bladder, without the use of adhesive tape. The catheter should be changed monthly.

3. **Vesicostomy** is a surgically formed fistula between the bladder and the abdominal wall. The bladder wall is sutured to the skin and the stoma is set in the midline just above the pubis. A vesicostomy appliance is applied over the stoma and is usually connected to collecting tube and bag. A nurse with special training or experience in ostomy appliances should be consulted for initial problems and maintenance.

The advantage of a vesicostomy is the elimination of an indwelling foreign body in the bladder. The disadvantage is that the bladder can contain a large volume of residual urine. Depending on the urologic procedure, the ostomy site may be predisposed to hair growth, which acts as a nidus for calculus formation. Cystoscopy is sometimes necessary to clean the bladder.

4. **Supravesical urinary diversion** is rarely indicated but can be critical in the face of progressive deterioration of the upper urinary tract in a patient with a neurogenic bladder. Direct cutaneous ureterostomy requires a stoma device. The "Bricker" ileal-cutaneous ureterostomy consists of a well-vascularized, isolated section of ileum that has been surgically interposed between ureters and skin. The "ileal loop" requires a stoma device and can be complicated by stomal erosion, stricture at the level of the skin, rectus abdominis, or ureteral anastomosis in the ileal loop. Serious infection and reflux may occur. There are other methods of surgical diversion.

UROLOGIC CONSULTATION

Other methods of diversion, augmentation cystoplasty, implanted external sphincters, and electrostimulation may be performed, but an initial consultation should always be sought from an experienced urologist. Not all urologists have an interest in the neurogenic bladder. The urologist should have a full understanding of the patient's physical disability, the natural history of his or her type of neurogenic bladder, and a working relationship with other health professionals involved in the patient's rehabilitative management.

REFERENCES

Boyarsky S, Labay P, Hanick P, Abramson AS, Boyarksy R: Care of the Patient with Neurogenic Bladder. Boston, Little, Brown, 1979.

Bradley WE, Timm GW, Scott FB: Innervation of the detrusor muscle and urethra. Urol Clin North Am *1*:3, 1974.

Kiviat M, Zimmermann T, Donovan WH: Sphincter stretch, a new technique resulting in continence and complete voiding in paraplegics. J Urol *114*:895, 1975.

Krane RJ, Siroky MB: Clinical Neuro-Urology. Boston, Little, Brown, 1979.

Raz S: Pharmacological treatment of lower urinary tract dysfunction. Urol Clin North Am *5*:323, 1978.

11

STOOL INCONTINENCE AND THE NEUROGENIC BOWEL

Lesions of the brain, spinal cord, or primary motor unit can result in fecal incontinence. There are three types of neurogenic bowels. **Uninhibited** type is due to a cortical or subcortical lesion in which mental awareness is impaired. Patients exhibit urgency or uninhibited defecation. **Reflex** type is due to lesions of the spinal cord. Sensory feedback from the rectum and cortical control over the anorectal mechanism are lost. The anal sphincter is spastic. Rectal emptying occurs reflexively when feces move into the rectum. **Autonomous** type can result from lesions of the conus medullaris or cauda equina in which the rectum and anus are denervated. There may be continuous expulsion of soft stool with relative retention of hard stool.

In a disabled patient, however, stool incontinence can occur as a result of gastrointestinal inflammatory disorders or fecal impaction. **Situational** incontinence can happen when a disabled person cannot reach the toilet or commode in time to evacuate.

COMPLICATIONS

The consequences of recurrent fecal incontinence from a neurogenic bowel can be devastating. The perineal skin may become macerated and predisposed to pressure sores, particularly over the ischial tuberosities and coccyx. A soiled perineum increases the risk of bladder infection in the presence of a neurogenic bladder, with or without the use of a catheter. Embarrassment, rejection, self-degradation, and withdrawal can characterize the disabled patient with a poorly managed neurogenic bowel. Chronic fecal incontinence can be symptomatic of widespread failure of the patient to follow recommendations.

PREPARATION FOR BOWEL PROGRAM

A. Describe the **pattern** of fecal incontinence: amount, color, consistency, odor of stool; frequency, time of day, relationship with meals; and association with body position, activity, sleep, and medication.

B. **Diet and fluid** history may reveal specific food items that "upset the stomach" and aggravate incontinence. A formal dietary history may be recommended to obtain data. The average amount of daily fluid intake is useful.

C. Inquire about **home remedies,** such as over-the-counter laxatives, enemas, diapers, perineal pads, and diet. Find out the patient's indications or reasons for using these remedies.

D. The method of **toileting** should be understood. Is a bedside commode used? Is the toilet accessible? Can wheelchair transfers take place safely? Is the height of the toilet seat adequate? What is the situation at school or work?

E. What is the **physical capability** of the patient? The answer requires knowledge of what the patient has demonstrated and often a physical examination of the patient's musculoskeletal system. How independent is sitting, transfer, standing, or walking? How much hand function does the patient have? Can the patient insert a rectal suppository, wipe the perineum, flush the toilet, wash the hands, hold a goose neck mirror, and dispose of equipment? To what extent have other people been directly involved in toileting the patient?

F. **Psychologic** factors are important to screen. Does the patient have a learning or emotional problem? Can the patient communicate? Does the patient perceive the fecal incontinence as a problem? What hours or activities during the 24-hour day are more or less vulnerable to a bowel accident?

G. The evaluation of **complicated** patients may require consultative assistance by a rehabilitation-oriented nurse, physiatrist, physical therapist, or occupational therapist.

Goals of a bowel program: Avoid chronic constipation or fecal impaction; keep a clean perineum and healthy skin; maximize independent toileting or minimize attendant help; and achieve socially acceptable continence of stool.

HEALTH EDUCATION

The disabled person and family should be told of the medical, hygienic, social, and economic consequences of the neurogenic bladder and secondary chronic fecal soiling. Emphasize the success that most disabled people have had with bowel programs. Point out that stool continence is a prerequisite for optimal bladder and skin management.

DIET AND FLUIDS

Through proper diet and fluid intake, the use of bulk formers, softeners, and enemas can be minimized or eliminated for many patients. Daily fluid volume should be about 2000–3000 ml for most disabled adults. The total intake may be modified by fluid restrictions imposed by the management of the neurogenic bladder.

Disabled patients tend to drink poorly because their physical disability restricts them. A diet of foods with a high water content, such as vegetables and fruits, should be encouraged. Warm liquids taken before breakfast can greatly facilitate the gastrocolic and duodenocolic reflexes.

Erratic eating habits should be minimized. Regular, well-balanced meals should be encouraged. Strong cultural food beliefs and life styles should be acknowledged when dietary changes, additions, or subtractions of specific food items are recommended.

A nutritionist or dietitian may be requested to work with the patient and family on evaluating the diet and suggesting changes that have the greatest chance of acceptance.

INTRA-ABDOMINAL PRESSURE

Abdominal binders or exercises, or both, can improve a patient's ability to generate sufficient pressure on a Valsalva maneuver to defecate. Maximal daily physical activity alone will promote peristalsis and maintain muscle strength.

TIMING

Timing, regularity, routine, consistency, and scheduling are the cornerstones of sound bowel management. Changes in the patient's program should be implemented in steps, preferably over a 7- to 14-day period, before instituting the next change. For example, withdraw or add laxatives one at a time. The program should be consonant with the life style of the disabled person and family. Avoid authoritative, inflexible recommendations as to when defecation should take place.

The timing of actual evacuation of stool is selected on the basis of when the patient can carry out toileting activity and the period of the day when continence of stool is extremely important to the patient.

A patient may prefer an evening evacuation to avoid the inconvenience and rush during the early morning. If the patient, however, is at greater risk for incontinence 6–8 or more hours following the evacuation, an early morning evacuation may eventually be necessary to avoid the embarrassment of an accident during work, school, or recreation. Many patients maintain effective stool continence with an every-other-day or twice-a-week evacuation.

RECTAL SUPPOSITORIES

Glycerine suppositories mechanically irritate the rectum and stimulate mucosal secretions that lubricate the feces to fill the rectum. One suppository is sufficient. Two or more suppositories at the same time provide little or no additional benefit.

Alternatively, **bisacodyl suppositories** mechanically and chemically stimulate bowel motility and secretory lubrication. The suppository should come in direct contact with the rectal mucosa. Abdominal cramping may be experienced but, except in children, is usually well-tolerated. The rectal mucosa can be irritated. There is no evidence, however, of an increased incidence of proctitis or rectal neoplasms. A bisacodyl pill should not be used as a first line medication because of its highly variable reaction time. Some individuals believe that taking the bisacodyl pill at bedtime promotes peristalsis during sleep and increases the effectiveness of an early morning bowel program. The bisacodyl suppository should be prescribed by its generic name because of cost. Its response time is approximately 15–30 minutes.

ANORECTAL DIGITAL STIMULATION

The patient or attendant should glove a finger and lubricate it generously. The patient should assume a supine or lateral position in bed. The gloved finger is inserted slowly into the rectum and moved in a circular motion until the external sphincter feels more relaxed. Stimulation usually takes a full minute or two. Digital stimulation may be repeated once or twice every 10–15 minutes, depending on the response. The patient may sit on a commode or toilet or lie in bed. Defecation, of course, can be assisted by mechanical removal of feces in the rectum.

Autonomic dysreflexia can be precipitated by sudden rectal stretch by feces, enema, or digital manipulation in the patient with a spinal cord injury at T4–6 or above. Unlike the autonomic dysreflexic response from neurogenic bladder causes, the episodes usually subside spontaneously and rarely require intravenous antihypertensive medication. Topical anesthetic over the anal mucosa, generous lubrication, and prompt discontinuation of an evacuation procedure can effectively treat dysreflexia.

PADS

Pads, diapers, tissue paper, and cloth pieces have been used to prevent soiling of undergarments and to allow easier cleaning. Disposable paper diapers or pads can add considerably to the monthly cost of supplies but may be very useful during episodes of diarrhea, frequent stool incontinence, or perineal dermatitis.

ORAL PREPARATIONS

Laxatives may be categorized as osmotic agents (e.g., milk of magnesia), bulk formers (e.g., mucilose, bran, psyllium seed husks), lubricants (e.g., mineral oil, dioctyl sodium sulfosuccinate), and irritants (e.g., castor oil, bisacodyl).

Bulk formers, such as mucilose, can supplement a diet that is low in fiber and residue. They are usually bland and nonirritating. (Metamucil, psyllium hydrophilic mucilloid, is available in powder in 7-, 14-, and 21-oz containers.) Patients may take 1–3 rounded teaspoons q.d.–t.i.d. to help maintain soft, bulky stools. Proper fluid intake is important. If chronic constipation or impaction is suspected, the bulk former should be temporarily discontinued.

Stool softeners, such as dioctyl sodium sulfosuccinate (DOSS), can soften stools. The usual adult dose is 100–300 mg P.O. q.d.–t.i.d. It is available in tablets or capsules (50, 100, 120 mg) over the counter. Patients report abdominal cramps and gas with "excessive" amounts of DOSS, which actually acts as an irritant by blocking water absorption in the small intestine. The capsule is usually preferred to the bitter syrup.

Educate patients about the various over-the-counter preparations. Warn them that some brand name preparations cost considerably more than the generic forms. Discourage the use of preparations with a mixture of softeners, bulk formers, and stimulants.

ENEMAS

Enemas are most effective in evacuating the rectum and lower sigmoid colon for constipation or impaction. As a rule, enemas are not necessary for routine bowel programs. Some patients, however, do respond better to enemas on an infrequent, but regular, basis.

TYPICAL BOWEL PROGRAM

Wake up at 6 A.M. Take a teaspoon of mucilose in a full glass of water or juice. Drink warm liquids and eat a high fiber breakfast. Fifteen minutes after breakfast, insert a whole bisacodyl suppository while lying in bed. Perform a digital stimulation 10–15 minutes later. Sit on a padded commode chair or toilet seat. If there are no results, repeat the digital stimulation. It may be necessary to stimulate the rectum again in 10–15 minutes. If there is no spontaneous defecation, gently remove the fecal contents of the rectum. For a patient who is establishing a bowel program for the first time, it may be useful to keep a record of when the program begins, number of stimulations, results, and incontinent episodes.

The clinic, office, or public health nurse is often the best qualified health professional to assist a patient in implementing a bowel program. The nurse should be accessible by telephone. An occupational therapist or physical therapist can assess the patient's bathroom at home from the standpoint of architectural barriers, transfers, grab bars, safety, and effectiveness.

REFERENCES

Chapman WH, Hill ML, Shurtleff DB: Management of the Neurogenic Bowel and Bladder. Oakbrook, Ill, Eterna Press, 1979.

Dietrich S, Okamoto GA: Bowel programs for children with neurogenic dysfunction, a followup. Arch Phys Med Rehabil 63:166, 1982.

Gass DD: Bowel training. Geriatric Nursing 4:16, 1968.

Sister Kenney Institute Staff. Introduction to Bowel and Bladder Care. Minneapolis, Sister Kenny Institute, 1975.

Staas WE, DeNault PM: Bowel control. Am Fam Physician 7:90, 1973.

12

AUTONOMIC DYSREFLEXIA

Autonomic dysreflexia or hyperreflexia can occur in a patient with a spinal cord injury at T4–6 and above. An episode of autonomic dysreflexia can occur suddenly and dramatically. A pounding headache, profuse perspiration, vague discomfort, and skin blotches accompany hypertension and a fall in heart rate. Many episodes, however, are less conspicuous and may occur frequently within a day. The hypertension can be malignant and, if left untreated, can result in loss of full consciousness, seizures, visual disorder, apnea, and cerebrovascular accidents from subarachnoid or intracerebral hemorrhages. Death can occur.

A **noxious** stimulus from usually the neurogenic bladder or the bowel precipitates a massive sympathetic discharge that, in patients with a T6 or lower spinal lesion, is reversed by inhibition from the brain. A major sympathetic response is the constriction of the splanchnic arterial system, which contributes to a sharp rise in blood pressure. The baroreceptors of the carotid sinus and aortic arch stimulate the vagus nerves, which are unaffected by the spinal cord lesion, to slow down heart rate. This vagal response, however, is insufficient to affect the hypertension.

Autonomic dysreflexia should be regarded as an **emergency.**

ACUTE MANAGEMENT

A. **Sit** the patient upright.

B. **Eliminate** the noxious stimulus. Palpate the lower abdomen for an enlarged bladder. Inspect the catheter for kinks or plugs. If necessary, irrigate an indwelling catheter or catheterize the bladder. Carefully perform a digital examination of the rectum to rule out an impaction. However, it is usually not necessary to disimpact the rectum because contact with the mucosa of the anus and rectum can become a noxious stimulus in itself.

C. **Monitor blood pressure** every 5–10 minutes.

D. **Antihypertensive drugs.** Most cases of autonomic dysreflexia subside spontaneously or as a result of proper action at the bedside. When hypertension appears malignant, however, intravenous medication should be considered.

1. **Trimethaphan** (Arfonad) is a ganglionic blocker with peripheral vasodilatation. One ampoule (10 ml of 50 mg/ml) in 500 ml 5% dextrose in water can be administered intravenously at a rate of 0.1–1.0 mg per minute. Its tachyphylactic and anticholinergic side effects demand constant vigilance. Lowering of blood pressure usually occurs within 10 minutes.

2. **Hydralazine** (Apresoline) may be more available and 10–20 mg can be given by slow intravenous push. A response within 5 minutes usually occurs. A rise in blood pressure within 10–60 minutes may necessitate another dose.

3. **Pentolinium** (Ansolysen) is an alternative ganglionic blocker with similar adverse effects. Pentolinium 5–10 mg can be given as an intravenous push every 5–10 minutes.

4. **Diazoxide** (Hyperstat) has potent arteriolar vasodilation and can be given intravenously as a bolus of 100–300 mg under 10 seconds. Its water- and salt-retaining properties have led some physicians to infuse furosemide 40–80 mg intravenously 10–15 minutes before diazoxide.

The blood pressure should be monitored frequently for hypotension, in which the patient may complain of a headache, lightheadedness, and feeling flush.

CHRONIC OR RECURRENT MANAGEMENT

Fecal impaction, urinary tract infection, pressure sores, and indwelling Foley catheters are examples of noxious stimuli that can cause recurrent or chronic dysreflexia. Phenoxybenzamine or mecamylamine may be considered:

1. **Phenoxybenzamine** (Dibenzyline) is an alpha-adrenergic blocker. Phenoxybenzamine 20–60 mg per day in 2 or 3 divided doses can lower blood pressure, particularly in situations involving an "irritable" neurogenic bladder. Its full effect may take 2–3 weeks. Nasal congestion, miosis, and postural hypotension are possible adverse side effects. The drug comes in 10-mg capsules.

2. **Mecamylamine** (Inversine) is a ganglionic blocker prescribed at doses of 2.5–5.0 mg P O t.i.d. Possible adverse effects can involve the central nervous system: seizures, tremors, depression, disorientation, drowsiness, and weakness. It is excreted by the kidneys.

PREVENTIVE OR ANTICIPATORY MANAGEMENT

There are a number of procedures that may trigger a dysreflexic response. A plan of action should be discussed prior to its implementation. These procedures are as follows:

Bowel care: anorectal digital stimulation; rectal suppository insertion; enema.

Bladder care: indwelling catheter; intermittent catheterization; irrigation.

Diagnostic procedures: sigmoidoscopy; colonoscopy; barium enema; cystoscopy.

Laparotomy: Manipulation of the gastrointestinal and urologic tracts.

Labor: Uterine contractions, childbirth.

Clothing: Tight garments, bands, straps, shoes.

Consult a physiatrist, urologist, anesthesiologist, or obstetrician with experience in the management of autonomic dysreflexia. With current knowledge, its mortality and morbidity should be very low in well-managed patients with spinal cord lesions at T4–6 or above.

REFERENCES

Erickson RP: Autonomic hyperreflexia, pathophysiology and medical management. Arch Phys Med Rehabil *61*:431, 1980.

Kewalramani LS: Autonomic dysreflexia in traumtic myelopathy. Am J Phys Med *59*:1, 1980.

Kursh ED, Freehafer A, Persky L: Complications of autonomic dysreflexia. J Urol *118*:70, 1977.

13

SELF-CARE

Self-care skills refer to those abilities necessary for independent, personal needs, such as eating, toileting, dressing, undressing, grooming, and hygiene.

Activities of Daily Living (so-called ADLs) embrace a wide range of self-serving, independent activities at home, work, or school or in the community. These activities include homemaking, child care, schooling, recreation, hobbies, sexual relations, wheelchair transfers, and self-care.

An impairment in vision, hearing, intellect, or musculoskeletal function may influence the efficiency and effectiveness of self-care. Although most disabled people learn to compensate for their deficits, technical aids and special techniques may greatly enhance their abilities.

EVALUATION

Be specific with the patient and family about each of the self-care skills. A referral to an **occupational therapist** is usually indicated if one or more of the self-care skills is performed tediously, inconsistently, unsuccessfully, or with partial or total assistance.

The occupational therapist can screen each self-care skill and decide what further testing is necessary to elucidate the clinical problem. Gross motor skills (e.g., bed turning, sitting, transfers, balance, equilibrium reaction) can be assessed. Evaluation involves joint range of motion, sensation, muscle strength, endurance, and coordination, particularly of the upper extremities, head, neck, and trunk. It is important to assess hand function in terms of grasp, pinch, specific muscle testing, edema, pain, and standardized performance tasks. The evaluation of visual perception and eye-hand coordination is often required. A home visit is sometimes necessary to observe the patient carry out specific self-care tasks outside the clinic or office setting and to assess the premises for architectural barriers.

Throughout the evaluation, the occupational therapist observes the patient's ability to learn, concentrate, and complete tasks in terms of quality and quantity. Judgment, impulsiveness, distractibility, memory, passivity, dependency on others, understanding, and communication are also evaluated.

MANAGEMENT

Self-feeding and **eating** are the most basic self-care skills. The patient may benefit by any of the following: enlarged utensil handle for a weak grasp, utensil holder cuff for an absent grasp, plate with a rim or guard for extraneous hand motion, rocker knife with a curved blade for one-handed cutting, and mobile arm support for proximal arm weakness.

Dressing and **undressing** can be improved by adaptive clothing and dressing aids. For example, a hemiplegic patient should be taught to place the involved arm into the shirt sleeve first but to remove it last in undressing. One-handed technique for tying shoe laces can be taught. Velcro fasteners can replace buttons, snaps, zippers, or hooks. A stocking aid can facilitate donning and doffing of socks.

Toileting can be improved by a raised toilet seat, external toilet frames for sitting, grab bars, suppository inserts, and various urinary collection devices.

Hygiene and **grooming** may be aided by a bathtub bench and a shower extension nozzle. A small bristle brush with suction cups may allow denture or fingernail hygiene using one hand. Long-handled toothbrushes allow dental hygiene for a patient with limited joint range in the upper extremity.

Orthotics and **plaster casts** may be recommended to prevent joint deformity, to compensate for weak muscle groups, to stabilize joints, and to promote specific hand function. Many orthotic devices require the expertise of a certified orthotist.

Prosthetic or **artificial limbs** for the upper extremity are fabricated by certified prosthetists. The occupational therapist can work with the prosthetist in teaching the patient the wear, use, and care of the prosthesis. The patient may be taught to maintain proper skin care, joint range of motion, and strength affecting the short limb. The occupational therapist may recommend ways that the patient can compensate for the deficient limb with and without the prosthesis.

Environmental control systems offer patients an option to master the environment electronically. The target device can be a lamp, alarm, intercom, television, radio, page turner, door opener, or tape deck. Some systems may be fixed to a powered wheelchair tray, allowing the individual to control the wheelchair and the remote environmental receiver into which one or more target devices are plugged. The vast majority of patients, however, can use simple, durable, inexpensive devices that have become available through commercial outlets (e.g., Sears, Radio Shack).

The selection of a control switch depends on the patient's physical disability and motor control. The switch may be a toggle, button, treadle, lever, joy stick, pedal, or tube connected to a pressure transducer.

The physician or physical therapist may consult the nearest major rehabilitation center regarding the use of environmental control devices for a particular patient.

REFERENCES

Adapt Your Own Clothing. Office of Independent Study, Division of Continuing Education, University of Alabama, University, Alabama 35486.

Aids for the Ill and Disabled, Vocational Guidance and Rehabilitation Services, 2239 East 55th Street, Cleveland, Ohio 44103.

Chasin J, Saltman J: The Wheelchair in the Kitchen. Paralyzed Veterans of America, 7315 Wisconsin Avenue NW, Washington, DC 20014.

Clothing for the Handicapped. Sister Kenny Institute, Chicago Avenue at 27th St., Minneapolis, Minnesota 55407.

Convenience Clothing and Closures. Talon Consumer Education and Velcro Corporation, 41 East 51st Street, New York, New York 10022.

Functionally Designed Clothing. Vocational Guidance and Rehabilitation Services, 2239 East 55th Street, Cleveland, Ohio 44103.

Hodgmen K, Warpeha E.: Adaptations and Techniques for the Disabled Homemaker. Sister Kenny Institute, Chicago Avenue at 27th Street, Minneapolis, Minnesota 55407.

Hopkins HG, Smith HD (eds): Willard and Spackman's Occupational Therapy, 5th ed. Philadelphia, J. B. Lippincott, 1978.

Klinger JL: Self-Help Manual for Arthritis Patients. Also available is Flexible Fashions. Arthritis Foundation, 1212 Avenue of the Americas, New York, New York 10036.

Lowman EW, Klinger JL: Aids to Independent Living, Self-Help for the Handicapped. New York, McGraw-Hill, 1969.

May E, Hotte E, Waggoner NR: Independent Living for the Handicapped and the Elderly. Boston, Houghton Mifflin, 1974.

McCartney P: Clothes Sense for Handicapped Adults of All Ages. Also available are Dressmaking for the Disabled and How to Adapt Existing Clothes for the Disabled. Disabled Living Foundation, 346 Kensington High Street, London W14-8NS, England.

Men's Fashions for the Wheelchair Set. Leinenweber, Inc., Brunswick Building, 69 West Washington St., Chicago, Illinois 60602.

Physically Handicapped. Extension Service, US Department of Agriculture, North Carolina State University at Raleigh, Raleigh, North Carolina 27607.

Trombly CA, Scott AD: Occupational Therapy for Physical Dysfunction. Baltimore, Williams & Wilkins, 1977.

Warren CG: Introduction to systems and devices for the disabled, Chap 20, pp 682–698. In Redford JB (ed): Orthotics Etcetera, 2nd ed. Baltimore, Williams & Wilkins, 1980.

Wheeler VH: Planning Kitchens for Handicapped Homemakers. Institute of Rehabilitation Medicine, 400 East 34th St., New York, New York 10016.

Communication is the primary goal of speech and language. In physical disabilities due to lesions in the central nervous system, it is common to find impairment in speech and language, such as delayed development, aphasia, and dysarthria. Effective communication is a cornerstone of effective rehabilitation.

EVALUATION

The physician should be keenly aware of the possible deficits in speech and language when interviewing a patient with a physical disability. "Mild" deficits, in fact, may signify important problems in comprehension and expression.

A. After taking a history from the patient and a member of the family, a careful neurologic examination with emphasis on the cranial nerves should be done.

B. Utilize the same style and materials for screening speech and language. For example, select an item, such as a wristwatch, and probe the patient in the following manner: "Describe its function. Name it. Write down its name. Write down its function. Read this word, 'wristwatch.' Put the wristwatch on. Wind the wristwatch." Ask the patient a few yes/no questions about the wristwatch.

C. Minimize cues during the assessment. Avoid subtle facial or body language. Do not give hints, clues, or reminders.

D. Utilize the same set of questions, tasks, or items in following the patient's progress. For example, ask the patient to name the same set of five common objects, such as a pencil, spoon, block, safety pin, and wristwatch, during each testing session and record the accuracy of responses.

In the presence of a speech and language deficit, a speech pathologist should be consulted. Standardized and careful clinical testing can be carried out to identify the problem and to formulate goals for treatment. Centers for rehabilitation medicine can suggest the names of qualified speech pathologists nearest the patient's residence.

DELAYED LANGUAGE DEVELOPMENT

In normal development, a sequence of speech and language milestones appear in a child. At 12 months, 3 words are spoken;

18 months, 20 words; 24 months, 270 words; 36 months, 900 words; 48 months, 1540 words; and 60 months, 2070 words.

By 3.5 years, the sounds of b, p, m, w, and h have been mastered. S, z, r, wh, v, f, and l sounds usually appear by 7.5 years. All speech sounds have been learned by age 8 years.

The language component of the Denver Developmental Screening Test can be used as a guide to assessing speech and language in young children.

The following conditions are frequently associated with significant problems in speech and language: inherited, congenital, or acquired disorders of the central nervous system; cranial nerve dysfunction; mental retardation; hearing loss; emotional disturbance; deprivation; and major musculoskeletal deformity.

Even the very young child should be evaluated by a speech pathologist. Most public school districts have a communication disorder specialist or speech pathologist.

A letter of referral should include pertinent information, such as birth history, early development, physical disabilities, medication, seizure disorder, and socioeconomic environment at home.

DYSARTHRIA

Disturbances in muscle control and coordination of the speech mechanism result in dysarthria, which is not always associated with language deficits.

Neuromuscular disorders, cerebral palsy, multiple sclerosis, parkinsonism, cerebrovascular accident, and traumatic head injury may be associated with significant dysarthria.

Dysarthric **patterns** can be categorized as flaccid, spastic, ataxic, hypokinetic, or hyperkinetic. The inexperienced physician should refrain from placing a label on the patient's speech and should describe it in ordinary words.

The **intelligibility** of dysarthria varies widely. The speaking rate may be reduced only slightly with normal intelligibility. Some patients, however, may exhibit nonfunctional, unintelligible dysarthric speech.

Mildly dysarthric patients may need treatment to slow rate, alter rhythm, and change unusual stress patterns of speech.

For more moderately involved patients, the speech pathologist may work on basic sound production, rate, and coordination of breathing and speaking.

For the **nonvocal** patient, the speech pathologist may recommend the involvement of specialists in rehabilitation medicine, occupational therapy, physical therapy, clinical psychology, medical equipment, and microprocessor computers in order to develop a comprehensive plan of management.

For example, proper seating of the patient may mean modification of the patient's existing wheelchair. The control device for an electronic or computer communication device might involve a joy stick, button, treadle, pedal, or sip-and-puff tube.

The communication device for the nonvocal patient may be simple and inexpensive to construct. A board with letters, words, pictures, or symbols may sit on the patient's wheelchair lap tray. Complex communication devices, on the other hand, involve cathode ray tubes (CRT), keyboards, ticker tapes, voice synthesizers, and flashing cursors on an electronic display panel. Highly specialized speech pathologists in this field are usually associated with major rehabilitation centers.

For the **family** of the dysarthric patient, the physician may suggest that normal conversation be used, unless the dysarthric person has a hearing or language impairment. The dysarthric person should slowly repeat the missed segment of conversation. If writing is easier in some social situations for the dysarthric person, a pencil and pad should be carried at all times.

ACQUIRED APHASIA

After language has been learned, brain injury may result in aphasia, or the impairment in language understanding and expression. Aphasia affects all processes of language, including listening, reading, speaking, and writing.

Fluent aphasia is characterized by effortless, well-articulated speech with normal rhythm and stress patterns. However, nonspecific words or words devoid of meaning are heard. Jargon or nonsense words may appear in fluent aphasia.

Nonfluent aphasia is characterized by limited speech, which is uttered slowly and with great effort. Poor articulation of words may occur. Speech may be telegraphic. For example, the patient may substitute "pencil write" for the complete grammatical phrase "A pencil is used for writing."

Because of the complexity of language, speech pathologists have begun to replace older terms, such as expressive aphasia, receptive aphasia, Broca's aphasia, and Wernicke's aphasia.

The common causes of aphasia usually involve damage to the dominant hemisphere. In 90% of people, the left hemisphere is dominant and houses the "centers for language." Eighty-five percent of acquired aphasia is caused by cerebrovascular accidents. Tumors, infection, encephalopathy, and head trauma account for the other causes of aphasia.

The speech pathologist screens the aphasic patient by careful evaluation of hearing, speaking, reading, and writing. For adults, standardized tests are available: Minnesota Test for Differential Diagnosis of Aphasia (Schuell, 1965), Boston Diagnostic Aphasia Examination (Goodglass and Kaplan, 1972), Porch Index of Communicative Ability (Porch, 1967), and other selective or comprehensive assessment tools.

The approach to the patient with aphasia is eclectic. The speech pathologist usually suggests the following: When auditory comprehension is reduced in the patient, others should use short sentences, gestures, and situational cues. The environment for communication should ideally be calm and quiet. The patient should be given time to respond. Hurried conversation should be avoided. The attention of the patient should be secured before conversation begins. Others should speak slowly and use natural pauses. An aphasic patient may be effective at pointing toward written words or phrases but be ineffective at writing.

REFERENCES

Beukelman DR, Yorkston KM: Speech and language disorders, Chap 5 pp 102–123. In Kottke FJ, Stillwell GK, Lehmann, JF (eds.): Krusen's Handbook of Physical Medicine and Rehabilitation, 3rd ed. Philadelphia, Saunders, 1982.

Bollinger RL, Wauth PF, Zatz AF: Communication Management of the Geriatric Patient. Danville, Illinois, Interstate Printers and Publishers, 1977.

Johns DF (ed): Clinical Management of Neurogenic Communication Disorders. Boston, Little, Brown, 1978.

Vanderheiden GC (ed): Non-Vocal Communication Resource Book. Baltimore, University Park Press, 1978. Bibliography of other literature is available from Trace Center, 314 Walsman Center, 1500 Highland Avenue, Madison, Wisconsin 53706.

Vaughan VC, McKay RJ, Behrman, RE (eds): Textbook of Pediatrics, 11th ed, pp 132–159. Philadelphia, Saunders, 1979.

15

NUTRITION

Patients with musculoskeletal disabilities are at risk for nutritional disorders. The primary physician should be alert to treatable or preventable nutritional complications. The nutritionist can work with the referring physician in evaluating and identifying deficits and, importantly, teaching the skills to correct them. Because national nutritional standards for specific physical disabilities have not been established, the physician and nutritionist should pool resources to arrive at a reasonable plan for the patient.

Numerous factors influence the nutritional condition of a patient: inadequate income to buy nourishing food; inability to shop, prepare meals, or eat; impairment in chewing and swallowing; low or high satiety; recurrent gastroesophageal reflux; abdominal cramping; chronic obstipation; and recurrent medical illness.

Adverse effects of medication, an imbalance between caloric output and input, and an ineffective bowel program may also influence a patient's status.

Psychologic factors are important. Depression, for example, will suppress appetite. Spouses, parents, or siblings may express their kindness or absolve their guilty feelings by excessive feeding, desserts, snacks, and "surprises" in the form of calorie-dense foodstuffs. For some severely disabled patients, control over eating may be one of the few activities by which the patient derives immediate gratification and exercises independent motor control.

EVALUATION

Weight is a sensitive indicator of changes in the patient's nutritional status. For the outpatient, weight should be obtained every 6 months. For a hospitalized patient in rehabilitation, weekly weighings are desirable. Special arrangements may be worked out to have the moderately to severely disabled patient weighed on a wheelchair or freight scale. Ideal body weight is only a guide, not a goal, for the patient with a disability. For children, standardized graphs should be plotted to follow the relative rate of growth.

Height or length is difficult to obtain in a patient who develops significant contractures of the spine, hips, knees, or ankles. The use of a stadiometer is often unsatisfactory. Reasonable estimates from arm span may be obtained in patients without shoulder or elbow contractures. Premorbid height and weight are important baseline data in comparing postdisability trends in linear or weight growth.

Other anthropometric measures, such as midarm circumference, are inadequately standardized and have specialized interpretative value for the nutritionist.

Laboratory tests include a hemoglobin/hematocrit, serum albumin, total protein, and specific vitamin or mineral analysis when indicated. Calcium, phosphorous, electrolytes, blood urea nitrogen, serum creatinine, liver function tests, amylase, and blood pH, for example, should be ordered by the physician as the patient's clinical condition dictates. Creatinine height index, 24-hour urea excretion, and other similar tests may clarify a patient's nutritional status in selective cases.

Dietary history should be recommended for patients who have a significant nutritional problem. A 1- to 3-day dietary diary or history can analyze the patient's choice of food items and total intake (calories, protein, fat, carbohydrates, vitamins, minerals, trace elements, and "supplements").

Feeding, chewing, and swallowing may be observed by a trained speech pathologist or occupational therapist. In some cases, cinefluoroscopy of swallowing and gastroesophageal activity may be needed to document dysphagia, gastroesophageal reflux, or inflammation.

MANAGEMENT

Setting nutritional goals should involve the patient and family. The goals should be re-evaluated periodically. Improvement should be generously applauded.

The physician should avoid lists of nutritional "do's" and "don'ts," unless preceded by careful explanation. Brief, glib comments at the end of a clinic visit seldom benefit the physician-patient relationship and devalue the importance of nutrition.

The disabled patient is vulnerable to dietary fads and is largely influenced by family and culture. The merits and potential harm of a "new diet" should be discussed in a nonjudgmental, objective, direct, and open-minded fashion. Harsh ridicule, opinionated remarks, and ignoring inquiry are likely to be counterproductive for the physician.

Many disabled patients depend on other people to help with shopping, cooking, or feeding. Dietary management should involve these significant others if changes are to occur at home, work, or school.

The nutritionist may recommend any of the following as goals: reduce weight; increase weight; prevent obesity; alter total caloric intake; drink more fluids; improve the intake of calcium, iron, trace elements, or vitamins; increase the proportion of protein; reduce simple carbohydrates; increase complex carbohydrates.

A change in the texture, taste, temperature, appearance, and quantity of food entering the mouth; the technique of placing a spoon in the mouth; the position of the patient's head, neck, and trunk during eating; choice of snacks; regularity of meals; and habits in shopping, preparation, and eating at the table are other possible recommendations.

The occupational therapist may recommend special utensils, cups, plates, and knives that compensate for the patient's physical disability. A balanced forearm "feeding" orthosis may be useful to a patient with weak upper extremities. A kitchen evaluation may be suggested to pinpoint problems in meal preparation, safety, efficiency, and adaptive equipment. A home visit may reveal architectural barriers. Adaptations of counter height, shelves, and drawers may make a considerable difference, particularly for the patient in a wheelchair.

REFERENCES

Dobie RA: Rehabilitation of swallowing disorders: Am Fam Physician 17:84, 1978.
Newmark SR, Sublett D, Black J, Geller R: Nutritional assessment in rehabilitation unit. Arch Phys Med Rehabil 62:279, 1981.
Peiffer SC, Blust P, Leyson JFJ: Nutritional assessment of the spinal cord injured patient. J Am Diet Assoc 78:501, 1981.

16

BEHAVIOR AND CHRONIC PAIN

A well-adjusted disabled person has learned behaviors that occur within the limits of his or her current physical, intellectual, and emotional capabilities. These behaviors are likely to result in successful life experiences.

The adjustment to disability involves the practice of behavioral skills repeatedly. For example, the disabled person learns to manage his or her neurogenic bladder and urinary incontinence in the community, away from home.

The process of adjustment varies and is **not a sequence of stereotypic stages** following the acquisition of a disability, such as a spinal cord injury and paraplegia. There is little empirical evidence to support the notion that adjustment proceeds in an orderly fashion and that the patient must go through each phase in order to attain full adjustment.

The **best predictors of long-time adjustment** are the person's psychosocial functioning prior to the onset of disability and his or her current social support.

The degree or severity of disability is not often a reliable indicator of optimal adjustment. A severely disabled person may resume work and family responsibilities well, whereas some mildly disabled people fail to attain independent living. Their failure to adjust may be partly due to persistent depression, chronic pain, inappropriate expectations, and other important influences.

EVALUATION

When interviewing the patient, the physician should pay attention to the patient's coping behavior in the past related to school, home, job, recreation, marriage, and community.

Ask about specific periods of stress, such as military service, divorce, death in the family, dismissal from work, poor grades in school, losing a competitive game, and prolonged illness.

Examine the patient's current status in terms of cognition, daily activities, significant others, economic resources, and community services. For example, sample an average weekday and weekend. Ask about how the day begins and ends.

Find out what the patient's personal goals are for education, work, and avocation. Determine if they differ from institutional goals for the patient.

Consultation with a clinical psychologist in rehabilitation may be sought. Trained counselors in vocational rehabilitation, social work, and physical disability may be important in assisting the patient.

Standardized psychologic tests may be recommended. The Wechsler Adult Intelligence Scale (WAIS), the Halstead-Reitan Neuropsychologic Assessment Battery, and the Minnesota Multiphasic Personality Inventory (MMPI) are often ordered. The interpretation of these tests, however, should be done by a psychologist who is thoroughly familiar with the specific physical disability.

More compehensive evaluations are recommended on an individual basis.

INDICATIONS FOR PSYCHOLOGIC CONSULTATION

A. The patient's **goals appear inconsistent** with his or her current level of physical, intellectual, and emotional functioning. For example, a C5 complete quadriplegic patient insists on becoming a heavy manual laborer. A person with a right hemispheric cerebrovascular accident maintains that he or she will return to bus driving.

B. The patient appears **reluctant to assume greater self-reliance** and, as a consequence, generates excessive stress on other family members. For example, a patient disabled by stroke is capable of walking with a cane and orthosis but insists that the spouse quit work, stay at home, and service him or her.

C. The patient demonstrates **self-destructive behavior despite admonishment to stop.** For example, the patient abuses alcohol, illicit drugs, or prescribed medication. The patient eats voraciously despite increasing problems with obesity.

D. The patient shows **classic signs of anxiety, depression, or other emotional problems.** For example, the patient exhibits insomnia, poor appetite, agitation, uncontrolled outbursts, and deterioration in social relationships.

E. The patient shows a **level of activity well below previously demonstrated physical capabilities.** For example, a patient with a mild musculoskeletal problem spends a lot of time in bed, complaining of pain. Sometimes, the patient chooses an activity that is well below his or her intellectual capability. The patient may be unable to cope with the burden of the newly acquired disability and the stress of the previous job simultaneously. Psychologic therapy may not be necessary. It is quite possible that this patient will become sufficiently proficient at managing the disability and develop the self-confidence necessary to return to the previous level of intellectual activity.

F. The patient has **counterproductive, unrealistic, underachieving, or unclear goals** regarding areas such as education, training, employment, and family.

PARTICIPATION

Involve the patient in decision-making. Point out choices or options. Keep the patient informed of plans for rehabilitative, medical, or surgical management. Consider marital therapy, biofeedback, relaxation exercises, and assertiveness training as ways to teach the patient how to deal with stress.

CHRONIC OPERANT PAIN

Pain is considered chronic in nature when it has persisted 6 months or longer or has recurred as a problem of long standing, or both. There are two kinds of classic pain.

Respondent pain refers to pain with a clearly identifiable and active organic source. Such pain, however, may not always respond to medical or surgical treatment.

Operant pain refers to pain with the following characteristics: It may have an identifiable organic cause. The active organic pathology, however, cannot be clearly indentified. The patient receives some forms of positive reinforcement or secondary gain.

Examples of positive reinforcement are as follows: Disability or monetary compensation; attention and concern from family, friends, spouse, physicians, and other significant people; attention waxes and wanes with the results from escalating doses of analgesics, especially narcotics; repeated requests for injections of medication to relieve pain are made. Patients with operant pain behavior will often avoid activities (e.g., stressful job, manual labor, housework, sex, school) that the patient perceives as unpleasant or as highlighting his or her inadequacies.

CLINICAL INDICATIONS FOR OPERANT PAIN EVALUATION

A. **Surgery.** Multiple operations aimed at pain reduction have failed. Patient insists on surgery despite clinical findings and recommendations to the contrary.

B. **Medical treatment.** Vigorous pain treatment has failed to produce reduction in pain within 6 months. Patient compliance with previous treatment has been inconsistent.

C. **Relief.** Quick, short-term relief from pain for periods of usually less than 2 months, subsequent to **new** treatment (e.g., heat, cold, transcutaneous electrical nerve stimulation, massage, medication), is soon replaced by pain at levels experienced prior to treatment.

D. **Medication.** Patient possesses several prescriptions for analgesics, sedatives, hypnotics, relaxants, or tranquilizers from several different physicians. The patient **escalates** the use of medication toward **full addiction.**

E. **Activity.** Daily activity is **low.** The patient is totally debilitated.

F. **Interpersonal** and **sexual relationships** have suffered.

CHRONIC PAIN PROGRAMS

The presence of one or more of the previous characteristics should prompt early consideration of a referral to a pain clinic. Most of these clinics offer comprehensive diagnostic, evaluative, and treatment services. The team may comprise a psychologist, physiatrist, anesthesiologist, neurologist, neurosurgeon, orthopedic surgeon, physical therapist, occupational therapist, vocational counselor, and social worker.

For some patients with chronic pain, an inpatient program may be recommended in order to bring about prompt control over the patient's total environment. The program should manage the patient's use of medication, daily activity, exercise, and diet. Social reinforcement for operant pain behavior should also be tightly managed with the cooperation of family and friends.

REFERENCES

Family doctor versus chronic pain. Patient Care *12*(14), 1978.

Fordyce WE: Behavioral Methods for Chronic Pain and Illness. St. Louis, CV Mosby, 1976.

Grzesiak RC: Chronic pain, a psychobehavioral perspective, Chap 8, pp 248–300. In Ince LP (ed): Behavioral Psychology in Rehabilitation Medicine, Clinical Applications. Baltimore, Williams & Wilkins, 1980.

Marinelli RP, Dell Orto AE (eds): The Psychological and Social Impact of Physical Disability. New York, Springer, 1977.

Treischmann RB: Spinal Cord Injuries: Psychological, Social and Vocational Adjustment. New York, Pergamon, 1980.

17

CONGENITAL AND CHILDHOOD-ACQUIRED DISABILITIES

The field of pediatric rehabilitation combines the functional approach of rehabilitation with the elements of growth and development in pediatrics. Clinical strategies must consider the child's developmental age as well as chronologic age. A great disparity may exist between them.

The primary disability under discussion is physical in nature. Mental retardation, blindness, and deafness alone deserve special discussion and are beyond the scope of this chapter. The more commonly encountered physical disabilities are as follows: major birth defects (myelomeningocele, limb deficiency, arthrogryposis), cerebral palsy, neuromuscular disorders (muscular dystrophy, poliomyelitis, polyneuropathy), acquired disabilities (spinal cord injury, brain injury, trauma to the limbs), and arthritides.

PRIMARY CARE

Many disabled children have complex or rare clinical problems that appear seemingly impervious to conventional treatment. Many families find their way to medical centers specializing in their child's disability. Primary care, however, is often lacking among high intensity, subspecialized, tertiary management. Clearly, there is a role for primary care.

Because of the child's physical disability, fundamental pediatric child care is often overlooked. The physician should perform the following: Immunize fully. Screen blood pressure, vision, hearing. Insist on routine dental care and daily oral hygiene. Obtain weight and linear measurements at recommended intervals for infants and preschoolers and no less than once annually for older children. Plot data on the NCHS Physical Percentiles Growth Charts (Courtesy of Ross Laboratories). If a child has contractured hips, knees, ankles, or spinal deformities, use maximal arm span as a crude measure of linear growth.

Obtain annual hemoglobin/hematocrit, urinalysis, urine culture, and other appropriate laboratory tests. In high-risk populations, tuberculosis skin tests should be performed every year.

Intercurrent, superimposed illnesses do occur in disabled children and may be unrelated to the physical disability. Complaints of illness should not be reflexively attributed to the physical disability.

The primary physician can develop and maintain a health care system for the child.

REHABILITATIVE GOALS

Intervention should facilitate the child's development, not impede it. Because parental dependency is an early, natural consequence of severe disability, parents should be made aware of this psychodynamic tendency. The conceptual differences between chronologic and developmental ages require frequent discussion with families. The use of medication, orthoses, therapy, and home programs for exercises should be supported if they appear to improve the child's function, prevent secondary complications, and enhance the child's development. "Treatment for the sake of treatment" should be discouraged.

The emotional, social, psychologic, and economic cost of rearing a disabled child can be very burdensome. The primary physician should screen the family for potentially serious psychosocial pathology. A few examples of an unhealthy parent-child relationship are as follows: infantilizing parenting; conspicuous silence of father or mother during office or clinic visits; evidence of physical abuse or neglect; alcoholism, drug abuse, unemployment, wife battery, transient residencies; vitriolic comments made toward health professionals; preoccupation with procuring "more" equipment, "more" surgery, "more" therapy for vaguely stated goals; chronic noncompliance or poor follow-up.

IMPAIRED MOBILITY

The goal of mobility should be safe, functional, independent ambulation. As a general rule, however, if a child has not achieved this goal within the home by age 7 years, it is unlikely, but not impossible, that the child will ever learn to walk independently. The physician should understand how extensive bracing, rigorous exercises, and multiple operations may deprioritize learning other important survival skills (e.g., self-care, toileting, pressure sore prevention, transfers, communication, socialization with peers and family).

A wide variety of powered mobility devices is available for children as young as 24 months to locomote independently. Major vendors in durable medical equipment are aware of these various mobility devices. There is no evidence that powered mobility in these young disabled children "takes away the incentive to eventually walk." Light-weight, finely balanced, so-called sports wheelchairs for children may greatly facilitate independent manual locomotion in children with high paraplegia.

IMPAIRED COMMUNICATION

A child may have severe impairment in speech, writing, or conventional typing. Over the past decade, the field of augmentative communication has developed to meet the special needs of these children. The child may learn to become more expressive, productive, and efficient in communication in home, school, and community. This skill is critical for a long-term outlook on independent living, vocation, and recreation.

Rehabilitation centers for children or adults usually have specialists who can properly evaluate and prescribe the most appropriate augmentative communication device for the child.

IMPAIRED SITTING

For the child who is unable to walk, seating is important for survival. It provides the structural support for comfortable, safe sitting and upper extremity activities. Proper seating can minimize the effect of gravity on a scoliotic or kyphotic progressive curve of the back, the occurrence of ischial decubiti, and the development of muscle or joint contractures.

The desired activity dictates the kind of seating system. For example, a severely disabled child may need three or more different seating systems for activities related to car transportation, eating, classroom work, toileting, and locomotion. Solutions range from inexpensive safety car seats to costly customized adaptations to a powered wheelchair.

SELF-CARE SKILLS

The evaluation and teaching of dressing, undressing, grooming, hygiene, and toileting are often overlooked or ignored. Walking with orthoses and crutches, for example, may be quite dramatic and thus receive a higher priority over learning other skills that will improve independence. An occupational therapist should be consulted to teach parents and the child special techniques, suggest adaptive equipment, and follow the child's development.

TOILETING

Bladder and bowel control are critical for a child's long-term survival. Great effort should be made to attain urinary and fecal continence at or prior to the child's enrollment in school. Close follow-up is important and often involves a urologist and nurse specialist.

SCHOOL

Any infant who is visibly lagging in development should be recommended for enrollment in a reputable infant stimulation program. As the child approaches 4 or 5 years, parents should know about Public Law 94–142 (1977), which mandates that school districts provide handicapped children with the opportunity to maximize their learning experience. A physician or concerned health professional can file a written request for an evaluation to make the disabled child a "focus of concern" at school. This activates a comprehensive assessment and the formulation of an Individualized Educational Program (IEP). The primary physician is often requested by parents or school officials to describe the child's physical disability. In addition, formal physical, occupational, and speech therapy often require a physician's prescription.

Premature assumptions of the child's mental impairment should be avoided. For some children, periodic consultation by a pediatric developmentalist, child neurologist, orthopedic surgeon, physiatrist, or neuropsychologist may be appropriate annually.

LEARNING SELF-RELIANCE

If a disabled child "fails" to learn a skill or complete a task, function, or activity, the physician should consider the following explanations:

1. The physical disability limits the child. Or, the child lacks the physical capability to perform.

2. The child lacks the cognitive ability to learn the skill.

3. Active superimposed chronic or acute illness inhibits learning and performance. Obesity, progressive scoliosis, symptomatic hydrocephalus, obstipation, and pyelonephritis are examples.

4. Overdosage or adverse effects of medication, such as antiseizure or anticholinergic drugs, may be present. Conversely, undertreatment may allow a disease to manifest itself.

5. Proper teaching has not taken place. For example, the child may have been ill during teaching and training sessions; the health professional may have been inexperienced, impatient, or inadequately trained; or the intensity and period of teaching might have been inadequate.

6. The specific skill or task may be inappropriate, irrelevant, impractical, or unfeasible outside of the clinic or hospital setting.

7. The child receives secondary gains from being "helpless" or "dependent" on parents and siblings.

8. The family deliberately or inadvertently is unsupportive of reinforcing more self-reliant behavior at home. A parent may perceive the child's capability differently and therefore not expect the child to carry out a newly learned activity.

9. The skill may be developmentally inappropriate for the child and, if introduced later, may be learned well.

10. The family does not have the social, psychologic, or economic resources to create a stable, structured environment. Parents may simply lack basic parenting skills. Marital discord, child abuse,

unemployment, and alcoholism, for example, may be highly destructive.

11. Labeling a child as "a failure," "lazy," "unmotivated," "apathetic," or "retarded" is, unfortunately, all too often an explanation for a child's difficulty in developing greater self-reliance. These terms pigeonhole children and suggest little or no constructive remediation. Thus, the lack of learning becomes the child's "fault."

REFERENCES

Bleck EE, Nagel, DA: Physically Handicapped Children: A Medical Atlas for Teachers, 2nd ed. New York, Grune & Stratton, 1982.

Downey JA, Low, NL (eds): The Child with Disabling Illness. New York, Raven, 1982.

Letts RM, Fulford R, Eng B, Hobson DA: Mobility aids for the paraplegic child. J Bone Joint Surg 58(A):38, 1976.

Okamoto GA: The rehabilitation of musculoskeletal disorders, Chap 41. In Kelley VC (ed): Practice of Pediatrics. New York, Harper and Row, 1981.

Shurtleff DB. Myelodysplasia: management and treatment. Curr Prob Pediatr 10:1, 1980.

Siegel IM: The management of muscular dystrophy: a clinical review. Muscle and Nerve 1:453, 1978.

Straub RR: Orthopaedic aspects of dwarfism. Orthop Review 11:49, 1982.

Vignos PJ: Rehabilitation in progressive muscular dystrophy, Chap 19. In Licht S (ed): Rehabilitation and Medicine. New Haven, Elizabeth Licht, 1968.

Williams P: The management of arthrogryposis. Ortho Clin North Am 9:67, 1978.

II

INDEPENDENT LIVING

18

INDEPENDENT LIVING MODEL

Independent living for disabled people means self-reliance, meaningful work, good health, interpersonal relationships, and integration into the community. Medical rehabilitation is necessary but not sufficient for the attainment of independent living.

Services for independent living include the following: housing with minimal architectural barriers; attendants for assisting the disabled person in daily self-care and mobility; transportation available for school, work, recreation, shopping, and socializing; properly maintained adaptive equipment; training for specific skills; counseling in areas of mental health, finances, law, employment, advocacy, physical care, and recreation; and medical services.

The concept of independent living does not mean segregation, isolation, or institutionalization in the community. For example, housing projects for the handicapped do not promote social integration of disabled residents. The disabled person should be able to direct his or her life.

Transitional living usually implies a bridge between hospitalization and community integration. The transition takes place within a prescribed time period and is largely directed by professional staff.

Rehabilitation in a hospital is characterized by a patient or client relationship with the health professional. Living is institutionalized. The patient has limited decision-making. The intensity of services is partly determined by how "sick" or "disabled" the "patient" is at any given point in time. Admission and discharge are medically related.

ROLE OF THE PHYSICIAN

Provide **primary care.** Many physicians are reluctant to become involved with physically disabled patients. The clinical problems may be very complex. The reimbursement for professional services is often limited. The constellation of consultants may be complicated. The chronicity of the patient's disability does not give the physician the kind of personal satisfaction that the management of acute, episodic illnesses gives most physicians.

Assist the disabled person in seeking proper medical and surgical attention. Emphasize prevention and positive health habits. Discuss medical goals. Establish a working relationship with consultants.

Involve the disabled person in decision-making. Present options, alternatives, choices, and opportunity where possible and appropriate.

Direct the disabled person to community support groups or individuals who have successfully adjusted to their physical disabilities.

Support legislation, community programs, and services that serve disabled people.

REFERENCES

Archives of Physical Medicine and Rehabilitation. 60(10):433, 1979. Entire issue is devoted to independent living.

Bruck L: Access: Guide to a Better Life for Disabled Americans. New York, Random House, 1978.

Disability Rights Center, 1346 Connecticut Avenue NW, Washington, DC 20036.

Disabled Student Service Center, Resource Catalog for Independent Living. San Francisco, San Francisco State University, 1977.

Hale G (ed): The Source Book for the Disabled. Philadelphia, Saunders, 1979.

Laurie G: Housing and Home Service for the Disabled. Hagerstown, Harper & Row, 1977.

National Center for Law and Handicapped, 1235 North Eddy Street, South Bend, Indiana 46617.

President's Committee on Employment of the Handicapped, A Handbook on the Legal Rights of Handicapped People. Washington, DC, US Government Printing Office, 1977.

19

RECREATION, LEISURE, AND COMMUNITY INTEGRATION

The recreational therapist may play a pivotal role in the rehabilitative process, particularly in the setting of a comprehensive hospital or community program. Faced with a physical disability, the patient may learn from a recreational therapist how to best use his or her existing abilities in the pursuit of recreation, leisure, and integration into the community.

EVALUATION

The recreational therapist interviews a patient to understand where he or she "is coming from." Attitudes, values, opinions, interests, perceptions, personality, and participation in the rehabilitative process are explored. Previous education, hobbies, sports, jobs, and family activities are noted. Formal tests may be administered to construct a patient profile.

The patient's physical, emotional, and mental condition should be clearly understood by the therapist. Medications, orthotics, prostheses, walking aids, and mobility devices of the patient should be known. His or her ability to walk, sit, transfer, propel a chair, control a powered mobility device, use a toilet, prevent skin breakdown, talk, groom, dress, and eat, for example, also provide a basis on which to prescribe recreational therapy.

CATEGORIES OF ACTIVITIES

Following selective discussion about the patient with other members of the patient's rehabilitation team, there is a variety of different activities that may be recommended by the recreational therapist; for example, arts and crafts; music, dance, drama; horticulture; games; cinema; reading; community dining; and group or one-to-one discussions.

Community-based activities may include the following:

1. **Travel.** Taking a bus ride, visiting the airport terminal, learning about van or sedan transportation, negotiating in crowds, crossing busy intersections.

2. **Social.** Eating at a restaurant or drive-in, attending spectator events (e.g., sports event, circus, parade, concert, movie), window shopping, visiting a museum, borrowing books at a library, buying supplies at a pharmacy.

3. **Architectural barriers,** particularly over sidewalks, curbs, parking lots, elevators, stairs, doors, rest rooms.

4. **Shopping.** Grocery store, supermarket, shopping mall, specialty shop, department store; asking for assistance; handling money; budgeting; preparing for a meal or social event.

5. **Meeting the "public."** Dealing with stares, insensitive remarks, well-meaning offers to be "helpful"; recognizing when assistance is needed, asking for help from strangers; teaching companions how to be supportive; being assertive, not aggressive.

GUIDELINES

A. The disabled person should learn that there are alternatives to boredom, isolation, and depression. Recreation can provide him or her with important options in living productively.

B. As part of a large rehabilitative process, recreational therapy can positively reinforce the disabled person through success-oriented activities and supportive social interactions with others.

C. The recreational program should have the following characteristics:

1. Provide an opportunity for the person to practice newly acquired skills such as wheelchair mobility and communication.

2. Follow the interests of the person, not the preferences of the therapist.

3. The person's specific physical disability should not determine the activity but rather the form of any given activity.

4. Emphasis should be placed on solving problems in the present before moving to the higher level of planning for the future.

5. Effective travel skills are critical for successful community integration.

RESOURCES

Arts and Crafts

Association of Handicapped Artists, 1134 Rand Building, Buffalo, New York 14203.

Association of Mouth and Foot Painting Artists, Fl. 9490 Vaduz, Kasperigasse 7, Switzerland.

Handicapped Artists of America, 8 Sandy Lane, Salisbury, Massachusetts 01950.

National Committee of Arts for the Handicapped, 1701 K Street NW, Suite 801, Washington, DC 20006.

National Council for Therapy and Rehabilitation Through Horticulture, Mount Vernon, Virginia 22121.

National Institute on New Models for Community Recreation and Leisure for Handicapped Children and Youth, Recreation Education Program, University of Iowa, Iowa City, Iowa 52240.

Volunteer Service for Photographers, 111 West 57th Street, New York, New York 10019.

Sports and Leisure Activities

General

National Association of Sports for Cerebral Palsy, United Cerebral Palsy Association, One State Street, New Haven, Connecticut 06511.

National Consortium on Physical Education and Recreation for the Handicapped, 1201 16th Street NW, Suite 610E, Washington, DC 20506.

National Handicapped Sports and Recreation Association, Penn Mutual Building, 3rd Floor, 4105 East Florida Avenue, Denver, Colorado 80222.

National Institute on Special Recreation, 362 Koser Avenue, Iowa City, Iowa 52240.

National Wheelchair Athletic Association, 40-24 62nd Street, Woodside, New York 11377 or 2107 Templeton Gap Road, Suite C, Colorado Springs, Colorado 80907.

President's Committee on Recreation and Leisure, Washington, DC 20210.

Archery

National Archery Association, 2833 Lincoln Highway East, Ronks, Pennsylvania 17472.

Basketball

National Wheelchair Basketball Association, Office of Commissioner, 110 Seaton Building, University of Kentucky, Lexington, Kentucky 40506.

Bowling

American Wheelchair Bowling Association, 2424 North Federal Highway 109, Boynton Beach, Florida 33435.

Dancing

Wheelchair Square Dancing (30-minute cassette), Colorado Wheelers, 525 Meadowlark Drive, Lakewood, Colorado 80226.

Flying

Wheelchair Pilots Association, 1101 102nd Avenue N, Largo, Florida 33540.

Golfing

National Amputee Golf Association, 24 Lakeview Terrace, Watchung, New Jersey 07060.
National Amputation Foundation, 12-45 150th Street, White Stone, New York 11357.

Horseback Riding

North American Riding for the Handicapped Association, Route 1, Medland, Georgia 31820.

Marathon

National Wheelchair Marathon Committee, 369 Elliot Street, Newton Upper Falls, Massachusetts 02164.

Music

Music Services Unit, The Library of Congress, Division for the Blind and Physically Handicapped, Washington, DC 20542.

Skiing

National Amputee Skiers Association, 3738 Walnut Avenue, Carmichael, California 95608.
United States Ski Association, Handicapped Skiers Committee, 6832 Marlette Road, Marlette, Minnesota 48453.

Softball

National Wheelchair Softball Association, PO Box 737, Sioux Falls, South Dakota 51101.

Swimming

Project Aquatic Mainstreaming, PO Box 698, Longview, Washington 98632.

Tennis

United States Table Tennis Association, PO Box 815, Orange, Connecticut 06477.

Travel

Amtrak Public Affairs, Access Amtrak. Washington, DC, 1977.

Annano DR: The Wheelchair Traveler. Milford, New Hampshire, Annano Enterprises, 1977.

Architectural and Transportation Barriers Compliance Board, Access Travel: A Guide to Accessibility of Airport Terminals. Washington, DC, 1977.

Atwater MH: Rollin' On: A Wheelchair Guide to US Cities. New York, Dodd, Mead, 1978.

Funk D: Guidelines for Transportation for the Handicapped, Washington, DC, Hawkins & Associates, 1979.

Laus MD: Travel Instructions for the Handicapped. Springfield, Illinois, Charles C Thomas, 1977.

National Park Service, Access National Parks, Washington, DC, 1978.

Reamy L: Travel Ability—A Guide for Physically Disabled Travelers in the United States. New York, MacMillan, 1978.

Society for the Advancement of Travel for the Handicapped, 3600 Wilshire Boulevard, Suite 1230, Los Angeles, California 90010.

Weiss L: Access to the World, A Travel Guide for the Handicapped. New York, Chatham Square Press, 1977.

US Government Printing Office: Access National Parks—A Guide for Handicapped Visitors, Washington, DC, 1978.

An architectural barrier is any type of environmental restriction that interferes with efficient and effective functional movement. Stairs, street curbs, narrow bathrooms, high countertops, and compact automobiles are frequently encountered examples of architectural barriers.

An architectural barrier may impose restrictions on pregnant women, the elderly, able-bodied children, and otherwise healthy people who have a temporary disability, such as a fractured leg, as well as people with chronic physical disabilities, mental retardation, blindness, deafness, and poor cardiopulmonary endurance.

EVALUATION

The physician may recommend that a physical or occupational therapist visit the person's home to evaluate its accessibility. Similar evaluation may be recommended for school and the work place. The therapist usually has access to printed material on building codes, ramps, and community resources.

Common "Minor" Household Barriers

Doorway: high threshold; narrow, heavy door; round, tight knobs; door swings into the room. **Floor:** thickly padded carpet; shag rug; scatter or area rugs; slippery runners over steps or hallways. **Turning space:** tightly arranged furniture; door opens into the room. **Bathroom:** slippery tub floor; no grab bars; low toilet seat; cabinet below the sink. **Kitchen:** stove controls high or at the rear; out-of-reach cabinets and shelves; high countertop. **Bedroom:** low bed height; insufficient shelves; narrow entry into closet; high rod for hanging clothes.

WHEELCHAIR ACCESSIBILITY

The wheelchair model used widely in the United States has two large rear wheels and two front casters. It requires a turning space of 1.5 × 1.5 meters (5 × 5 feet), which may be reduced to 0.9 × 1.2 meters for more linear movement.

By sitting in a wheelchair, the average adult reduces standing height by one third, doubles his or her width, and limits arm reach to only 10–20 cm beyond the knees and feet.

In a home, architectural solutions do not necessarily entail expensive remodeling. For example, the arrangement and kind of furniture in a room can facilitate wheelchair mobility.

Entry and **egress**. Walkways should be 1.2 meters (4 feet) wide. Islands of raised or sunken stepping stones should be avoided.

Ramp gradient should rise about 2.5 cm for every 30 cm of length (1 in. for every foot). The steeper the gradient, the more useful handrails are. Use a nonslip, firm surface. Avoid ramp impediments rising over 1.25 cm (0.5 in.). Consider resting platforms measuring 1.5 × 1.5 meters (5 × 5 feet) at intervals of 9.0 meters (30 feet).

Doors should be 80 cm (32 in.) or more in width. Doorknobs should be placed no higher than 90 cm (36 in.) from the floor. Lever handles are easier to manipulate than round knobs. Eliminate door sills. Consider 30.0 cm (12 in.) high kickplates at the base of doors.

Stairways should have tactile warning signs and continuous, nonslip handrails. Avoid slippery runners.

Floors should be firm, level, and nonslippery. Avoid scatter or area rugs. Carpets with low pile and dense weave are preferable. Minimize padding and shag rugs.

Controls for lights, drapes, fire alarms, emergency power, and windows should be placed between 45 and 120 cm (18 and 48 in.) above the floor.

The **bedroom** should accommodate special equipment and supplies that are important for self-care. Adjust the bed height to facilitate wheelchair transfers. Closets should have wide entry, low hanging bars, and open shelves.

The **kitchen** should have a minimum clear space of 1.2 × 1.2 meters. Ideally, space under cabinets or counters should clear a wheelchair or have a toe space of 23 cm (9 in.) high and 15 cm (6 in.) deep. Counters may be 54 cm (22 in.) deep and 82 cm (33 in.) above the floor. Countertops are most comfortable 8–20 cm (3–8 in.) below elbow height. The stove should have low-set, front controls. Microwave ovens offer some advantage and eliminate the risk of reaching into a hot oven.

The **bathroom** is costly to remodel. The ideal space for maneuverability is similar to that for the kitchen. The sink should be fixed to the wall about 78–80 cm (31–32 in.) high. Equip the shower stall (90 × 90 cm) with a chair, grab bars, and flexible hose for the shower head.

Grab bars (80 cm [32 in.] high) should be anchored near the toilet seat and by the bathtub. Towel rods and soap dishes should not be used as rails. Tub benches and raised toilet seats may reduce the difficulty of transfers and improve safety.

The most suitable **automobile** for a disabled individual depends on many factors. For the independent person with paraplegia, a large two-door sedan does allow efficient wheelchair transfers and storage of the folded wheelchair in the back seat. An individual with quadriplegia in a powered wheelchair would benefit greatly from a van with a hydraulic lift.

REFERENCES

Catalogs and brochures for home health aids are available through Sears, Montgomery Ward, JC Penney, Abbey Medical, and many other companies.

Chasin J: Home in a Wheelchair. Paralyzed Veterans of America, 7315 Wisconsin Avenue NW, Washington, DC 20014.

Daniels M (ed): Ramps Are Beautiful. Center for Independent Living, 2539 Telegraph Avenue, Berkeley, California, 1982.

Foot SF: Handicapped at Home. Design Centre Book, Disabled Living Foundation, 346 Kensington High Street, London W14–8NS, England.

Kliment SA: Into the Mainstream: A Syllabus for a Barrier-Free Environment. National Easter Seal Society, 2023 West Ogden Avenue, Chicago, Illinois 60612.

Mace RL, Laslett B (eds): An Illustrated Handbook of the Handicapped Section of the North Carolina Building Code. Department of Insurance, PO Box 26387, Raleigh, North Carolina 27611, 1974.

National Center for a Barrier Free Environment, 8401 Connecticut Avenue, Washington, DC 20015.

Schweikert HA: Wheelchair Bathrooms. Paralyzed Veterans of America, 7315 Wisconsin Avenue NW, Washington, DC 20014.

Small R, Allan B: An Illustrated Handbook for Barrier Free Design, Washington State Rules and Regulations. Easter Seal Society Accessibilities Unit, 521 2d Avenue West, Seattle, Washington 98119, 1978.

Wittmeyer M, Barrett J: Housing Accessibility Checklist. Department of Rehabilitation Medicine, Seattle, University of Washington, 1980.

21

DRIVING AN AUTOMOBILE

Through experience and mechanical ingenuity, **adaptive driving** has afforded many physically disabled adults the opportunity to drive motor vehicles safely and effectively. The primary physician may play an important role in facilitating the process of evaluation.

Evaluation programs exist and can be contacted through the state Department of Motor Vehicles and Licensing. Most large rehabilitation centers have specialized evaluation programs.

PATIENT AS A CANDIDATE FOR EVALUATION

Using the following guidelines, the physician may consider a patient as a candidate for a driver's evaluation:

1. Patient expresses an desire to drive but tempers it with an acknowledgment of his or her mental, physical, or emotional limitations.

2. The patient's condition is improving or stable, not deteriorating. If the patient has a seizure disorder, drug compliance should be excellent and the history free of symptoms for more than 6 months. Patient should be under regular physician care.

3. The patient takes prescribed medication responsibly and conscientiously and is aware of potential adverse side effects.

4. Drugs or alcohol are not abused.

5. Patient has demonstrated responsibility in maximizing his or her abilities to be self-reliant. Toileting, skin care, and wheelchair mobility, for example, are performed competently.

6. Visual-spatial perception, communication, voluntary motor control, and reasoning appear potentially appropriate for safe driving.

7. Patient is rational and predictable, and takes criticism. Physically or verbally explosive, aggressive, hostile, or paranoid behavior should **not** be present. The patient should not have suicidal ideation or have recently attempted suicide.

8. Optimally, the family should be supportive and firm.

The physician should refer the disabled person who expresses a burning desire to drive but is viewed as a marginal candidate. Specific concerns, however, should be registered in the letter of referral.

PHYSICIAN REFERRAL

Although each program has its own procedures and forms for evaluation, the primary physician may expedite the process by submitting a letter of referral. It should contain statements relevant to the patient's driving capability or potential as perceived by the physician. The letter may include the following:

Physical impairment: its nature? etiology? progression? deformity? weakness? incoordination? endurance? **Vision:** acuity, peripheral fields, scanning. **Medication:** type of drug? side effects? reason for use? **Functional skills:** use of crutches? wheelchair? transfers? hand dexterity? prostheses? orthoses? sitting tolerance? muscle spasms? **Hearing:** deaf? hearing aid? **Communication:** dysarthric? **Psychologic:** problem-solving? impulsivity? distractibility? judgment? memory? confusion? agitation? hostility?

EVALUATION

In most driver-evaluation programs, the documentation regarding the applicant is thoroughly reviewed. An interview takes place. A functional examination is often required. Muscle strength, joint range of motion, endurance, coordination, reaction time, vision, and hearing may be selectively evaluated.

Laboratory evaluation may involve a mockup of a car seat and controls for driving. Transfers, sitting, manipulation of controls, and problem-solving are observed. Visual screening may include acuity, depth perception, peripheral fields, scanning, spatial relationships, and color discrimination.

The person may next be assessed in a training car.

ADAPTIVE DEVICES

The evaluation may result in specific recommendations for assistive devices or standard modifications, such as conventional power steering, power brakes, automatic transmission. **Hand controls** may be pull-push, twist-push, or right angle–push. The **steering** mechanism may have a spinner or other attachments, such as plain knob, latch, palm grip, tri-pin, driving ring, cuff, V-grip, or valve. **Transfer** devices include sliding boards, hooks, bars, loops, straps, or floor boards. Hooks or extensions may be used for brakes, turn signals, gear shifts, and parking. Pedals may have blocks. The mirror may be wide and full. **Seating** modifications may include safety belt, chest harness, or seat cushion.

THE VAN

A van may be ideally suited for certain severely disabled people who rely on motorized wheelchairs for locomotion. Lifts, wheelchair locks, and control panels designed for powered wheelchairs have greatly maximized independence in mobility for these individuals. High initial costs of the van should be weighed against the immediate and long-term benefits of community mobility.

ON-THE-ROAD EVALUATION

Depending on state regulations and the person's current license status, a learner's permit is usually necessary prior to on-the-road testing and training.

Standardized flow sheets give the evaluator and person an objective report on progress. The graduate of the training program may then proceed to the testing center of the state Department of Motor Vehicles and Licensing. Virtually all testing centers accommodate disabled people and try to assess driving competency objectively. The previous tester and trainer may provide invaluable information on the person's driving potential.

THE UNSAFE DRIVER AS A PATIENT

Until the state or federal government has passed legislation for reporting unsafe drivers, the physician, therapist, psychologist, and other health workers may become involved in a medicolegal dilemma with the patient who is medically assessed as unfit to drive a motor vehicle. If the patient is openly defiant and expresses an intent to drive a motor vehicle, the following guidelines for action should be considered:

1. Discuss the medical or psychologic limitations of the patient with him or her and the family. This task may be difficult when the issue is mental, emotional, or psychologic disability more than physical inability. The adverse effect of medication should be explained, if appropriate.

2. Obtain a signed statement from the patient or a family member that the discussion had taken place, the risks explained, and the negative recommendation about driving made.

3. For the incorrigible patient with an ineffective or contradictory family, the physician should consider a letter (return receipt requested) to a specific person in the state's Division of Motor Vehicles in addition, perhaps, to a telephone call.

4. Judgement, of course, must always be used. Consultation with an officer of the state medical association or an attorney versed in medical law may be desirable at any point.

REFERENCES

Driver Education for the Physically Disabled: Evaluation, Selection and Training Methods. Institute for Rehabilitation Medicine, 400 East 34th Street, New York, New York 10016.

Duncan DD, McDermott M, Peizer E: Automotive wheelchair lifts: development of standard criteria for their evaluation. Arch Phys Med Rehabil 59:437, 1978.

Handicapped Driver's Mobility Guide and Vehicle Controls for Disabled Persons. American Automobile Association, 1712 G Street NW, Washington, DC 20015.

Jacobs S: Reporting the handicapped driver. Arch Phys Med Rehabil 59:387, 1978.

Less M, Colverd ED, DeMauro GE, Young J: Evaluating Driving Potential of Persons with Physical Disabilities. Albertson, New York, Human Resources Center, 1978.

———Hand Controls and Assistive Devices for the Physically Disabled Driver. Albertson, Human Resources Center, 1977.

———Teaching Driver Education to the Physically Disabled. Albertson, Human Resources Center, 1978.

22

VOCATIONAL COUNSELING

INTRODUCTION

The disabled person is at a disadvantage in the usual working situation unless specific changes occur and allow for maximal function. This unique interaction between vocations and disabilities forms the basis for professional vocational counseling.

The prospect of proper training, education, and employment depends on many variables. The physically impaired person is most vulnerable to adverse trends in the economy and is, perhaps, the last to benefit from positive trends in employment. Nevertheless, there are many highly productive people with physical disabilities in the work force.

Visible and invisible disabilities. Visible disabilities are characterized by obvious physical impairment, walking aids, wheelchairs, and other specialized equipment. Cerebral palsy and paraplegia from spinal cord injury are visible disabilities. In contrast, invisible disabilities often have no overt stigmata, as in diabetes mellitus, heart disease, emphysema, renal disease, and epilepsy. Employers and employees tend to lower their expectations of people with visible disabilities and raise their expectations of people with invisible disabilities disproportionate to the person's true potential.

The physical disability may correlate poorly with the person's work potential. For example, paraplegia from spinal cord injury may be less disruptive for an engineer or accountant. An acquired amputation of a finger in a musician, however, may be devastating.

EVALUATION

The physician should be aware of **vocational counseling** as a specialized service. A counselor's clientele may have one of the following disabling conditions: paraplegia or quadriplegia from any cause (spinal cord injury, myelomeningocele); cerebral palsy; brain injury; amputation; chronic pain syndromes (neck, shoulder, arm, hand, back, leg, foot); limited cardiovascular endurance; cerebrovascular accident; progressive disorders (multiple sclerosis, parkinsonism, muscular dystrophy).

An arbitrary **gradient of physical work** has been utilized as a guideline in categorizing a person's capability. Sedentary work involves 4.5 kg of lifting; light work, 9.0 kg; medium work, 22.7 kg; heavy work, 45.5 kg; and very heavy work, 45.5+ kg. The intensity of sitting, standing, walking, carrying, pushing, pulling, bending, and climbing varies with each level of work. The physician may consider the patient's work potential in this manner.

A summary of the patient's medical history and physical examination is pertinent to the intake process. The vocational counselor may be a case manager or consultant from the state Department of Vocational Rehabilitation (DVR), state Department of Labor and Industries, private practice, or a comprehensive rehabilitation center. Vocational counseling may also be available in schools, colleges, technical training centers, and universities.

The basic evaluation involves a detailed interview and appropriate testing for interests, achievement, aptitude, and personality. The **interest inventories** compare the person's pattern of interests with the general and select populations. They should not be used to predict vocational outcome. Strong-Campbell Interest Inventory, Career Assessment Inventory, Minnesota Vocational Interest Inventory, and Kuder Occupational Interest Survey are examples of interest tests.

Aptitude tests assess the person's ability in specific areas of competence and are represented by the General Aptitude Test Battery, Differential Aptitude Test, SRA Primary Mental Abilities, Purdue Pegboard Test, Minnesota Clerical Test, and the Test of Mechanical Comprehension.

Personality tests may suggest clear patterns of behavior that might enhance or impede vocational pursuits. The Minnesota Multiphasic Personality Inventory (MMPI), Edwards Personal Preference Schedule, Sixteen Personality Factors Questionnaire, and the California Psychological Inventory are examples.

The vocational counselor may recommend further testing by a social worker, clinical psychologist, speech pathologist, occupational therapist, or a physical therapist. Consultation from a physiatrist, neurologist, orthopedic surgeon, cardiologist, pulmonologist, rheumatologist, and nephrologist may be sought.

MANAGEMENT

The **objectives** of vocational counseling are as follows: Evaluate the person's rehabilitative potential. Guide the person in the exploration and selection of a vocation. Assist the person in preparation, training, and placement. Help the person maintain employment.

A **work station** or trial work program may be offered at some urban medical and rehabilitative centers. It offers a simulated work environment to assess the person's ability to manage a job.

A **sheltered workshop** is designed to facilitate evaluation and train disabled people in a realistic job setting. The workshop may train the person for job placement outside the workshop. The program may have training and permanent employment programs under one roof. Eligibility, aptitude, physical competence, and productivity requirements vary. Often, a sheltered workshop is specific for a certain category of disability, such as blindness, deafness, cerebral palsy, traumatic brain injury, or mental retardation.

A major weakness of American vocational programs for disabled people is related to **built-in disincentives** to work. Disability-related incomes may be forfeited in the event the person finds gainful employment and surpasses the maximal allowance for gross personal income. The loss may involve comprehensive, government-funded health insurance. Problems with appropriate housing, public transportation, and attendant services at home create other serious barriers.

Each state has a **division of vocational rehabilitation** funded by the federal government to provide vocational services to disabled people. The age eligibility is 18–62 years. Services include evaluation, counseling, education, training, rehabilitation, and psychologic treatment. Specific services may be provided directly out of the DVR office or subcontracted to other agencies or practitioners in the community. The exact governing rules, regulations, and funding vary from state to state. The process of intake may be initiated by a physician's **letter of referral** to the nearest or central DVR office.

A counselor or case manager may be assigned to the person. An **Individual Written Rehabilitation Plan** (IWRP) is often developed, based on the person's specific disability, level of independence, and great rehabilitative potential. The person's primary physician is frequently asked to provide appropriate documentation and comment on the person's vocational abilities.

The **Workman Compensation Programs** are funded by state and federal governments and cover people who have sustained injuries related to the job. For example, a disabling acute and chronic low back pain due to manual labor at work makes the person eligible for program benefits under most circumstances.

Monetary compensation and awards for the specific disability (partial v. total; temporary v. permanent) distinguish the Workman Compensation Program from the DVR program. The physician may facilitate the person's intake by providing a letter of referral that details the degree of disability and prognosis. Judicial hearings may involve formal testimony or deposition by the physician in terms of estimating the degree of disability and prognosis.

Private sector programs are sponsored by large insurance companies that insure employers. These programs are similar to the state Labor and Industries Programs. The primary physician may initiate the referral for evaluation and counseling by fee-for-service vocational counselors. Many insurance plans for employers and health insurance policies lack vocational services.

REFERENCES

Athelstan GT: Vocational assessment and management, Chap 8, pp 163–189. In Kottke FJ, Stillwell GK, Lehmann JF (eds): Krusen's Handbook of Physical Medicine and Rehabilitation, 3rd ed. Philadelphia, Saunders, 1982.

Stolov WC, Clowers MR (eds): Handbook of Severe Disability. Washington, DC, US Government Printing Office, 1981.

Stolov WC, Hooks DL: Prevocational evaluation, Chap 9, pp 190–198. In Kottke FJ, Stillwell GK, Lehmann JF (eds): Krusen's Handbook of Physical Medicine and Rehabilitation, 3rd ed. Philadelphia, Saunders, 1982.

23

SEXUAL DYSFUNCTION

Sexual dysfunction is the loss of sexual performance at the previous or expected level of functioning due to physical impairment.

Physiologic dysfunction is usually due to a lesion in the neural pathways. As a result, a loss in erection, lubrication, ejaculation, or emission may occur.

Mechanical dysfunction may result from problems in positioning, as in arthritis, spasticity, flaccidity, and chronic pain; from lack of body motion, as in spinal cord injury, cerebral palsy, and brain injury; and from adaptive equipment, as in catheters, drainage bags, and body jackets, which interfere with sexual activity.

Social dysfunction involves poor sexual-social skills to attract a partner, as well as unhealthy societal attitudes toward the sexuality of disabled people.

Psychologic dysfunction is the inability of the disabled person or partner to accept changes in sexual functioning due to the disability.

MANAGEMENT OF PHYSIOLOGIC IMPAIRMENT

Loss of Erection and Lubrication

This loss is commonly seen in disabilities, such as spinal cord injury and myelomeningocele, which affect function of the upper and lower motor neurons. Erections may occur reflexively from tactile stimulation of the penis or from psychogenically induced stimuli, such as intellectual fantasy, anticipation, and visual imagery. Ninety per cent of upper motor neuron injuries are associated with adequate reflex erections. Twenty per cent of patients with lower motor neuron injuries at T12 or below achieve fleeting psychic-related erections.

A. Treatment for **inadequate lubrication** for the female is water-soluble jelly (e.g., K-Y Jelly).

B. Treatment of **inadequate erections** may involve a rubber band or condom at the penile base, which will reduce venous return and augment erections. The female partner may "stuff" the semierect penis into the vagina and attempt to improve blood flow into the penis by movement and a "milking activity" of the vaginal muscles. This technique of stuffing works only with partial erections and a coordinated partner.

C. Treatment of **absent erections** does not require any special intervention if the partner and the disabled person are satisfied with the use of hands, mouth, or other forms of stimulation. If the sexual relationship is successful **and** one or both partners would enjoy the added stimulation of an erection, a penile implant can be inserted. Presurgical counseling is necessary to prevent undue expectations. An implant cannot be expected to save a failing relationship.

There are basically **two options**: a semirigid **Silastic prosthesis** (Small-Carrion) can be fitted into both corpora cavernosa to provide a permanent partial erection. This is somewhat embarrassing for those with ambulatory ability but is not noticeable when the patient sits in a wheelchair. The prosthesis must be fitted well to prevent the major complications of protrusion out of the fascia and infection.

An **inflatable prosthesis** (Scott) is the other option. It is a pair of inflatable tubes that essentially replace the corpora cavernosa. These tubes are filled from an abdominal wall reservoir through valves in the scrotum. Mechanical failure, lengthy surgery, and high expenses limit its use.

Loss of Ejaculation

Ejaculation may be defined as forceful rhythmic expulsion of semen from the urethra, controlled by sacral spinal segments 2, 3, and 4. This loss may be seen in spinal cord injury, multiple sclerosis, polyneuropathy, and other disabling physical conditions. Only 1–5% of patients with upper motor neuron spinal cord injury have ejaculation. Ejaculation does not occur in patients with lesions of the lower motor neuron involving sacral segments 2, 3, and 4. Retrograde ejaculation may occur into the bladder.

There is no physiologic cure. Patients, however, should be counseled about the social adjustment to loss of ejaculation.

Loss of Emission

Emission is defined as the movement of semen and sperm from the vas deferens, seminal vesicles, and prostate into the urethra, controlled by the lower thoracic sympathetic neurons.

Loss of emission may be seen in spinal cord injury, multiple sclerosis, and polyneuropathy. Its prevalence in other disabling conditions is not known. In upper motor neuron spinal cord injury, about 1–3% of semen is expelled. In lower motor neuron lesions, the average amount of emission is 15–25%.

There are no known cures. The patient should be counseled for social adjustment to the loss of emission.

Loss of Fertility

In women, the normal return of ovulation usually occurs 1–6 months after the acute injury. In most disabling conditions, there is no loss of fertility. Depending on the social situation, the physician or associate may consider health education on birth control. Most lay people express surprise when they learn that physically disabled women can conceive and bear children.

In men, the fertility rate in spinal cord injury, complete and incomplete, is only 5%. Temperature control and blood supply to the testes are lost, although the pituitary-testicular axis is usually normal. Ejaculation and emission rates are low. Intercourse is infrequent.

There is no current treatment in men for infertility secondary to spinal cord injury. Experiments have been conducted in electro-ejaculation, but no practical intervention has been developed.

MANAGEMENT OF MECHANICAL DYSFUNCTION

Indwelling Catheters. In the disabled woman, the bladder catheter may be ignored. In the disabled man, the catheter may be folded under a well-lubricated condom.

Positioning Difficulties. The rear entry, side-lying position may be the best position for patients with arthritis or hip flexion contractures. A bolster between the knees may be necessary for patients with severe adduction spasticity or scissoring at the hips.

AUTONOMIC DYSREFLEXIA

In patients with spinal cord injury at T4–6 or above, orgasm may trigger a mild hyperreflexic episode. The disabled person should sit up and allow relaxation to take place gradually. The episode is almost always self-limiting and usually poses no hypertensive threat.

DRUG INTERACTION

Drugs may aggravate the impairment in physiologic functioning. Phenoxybenzamine hydrochloride (Dibenzyline) may cause bladder neck relaxation and retrograde ejaculation. Diazepam (Valium) may depress all reflex responses. Propantheline bromide (Pro-Banthine) may lessen erections and lubrication. Antidepressant and antihypertensive drugs may decrease sexual responses.

PSYCHOLOGIC AND SOCIAL ADJUSTMENT

Society views the disabled person as less able sexually and less intelligent. People are reluctant to become "involved," partly because of popular societal myths and superstitions. Architectural barriers may passively discourage social contacts and partner availability. The disabled person must have unusually high sexual-social skills to overcome these societal problems.

With the acquisition of disability, the previously able-bodied adult will experience an abrupt change in body image and sexual performance. Anger and depression usually accompany the loss of ability and may lead to a loss of sexual confidence and self-esteem. A fear of failure in sexual relationships often leads to further reduction in sexual activity.

Treatment should be directed at understanding the physiologic disability, relief of anger and depression, encouragement of sexual exploration, and, if appropriate, counseling on specific sexual-social skills.

Lack of communication frequently occurs between sexual partners when the newly acquired disability produces major changes in the person's physiology, sensation, and movement. Counseling is often very helpful in assisting partners to deal with the sexual problem in a constructive, open, sensitive way. For example, "I would like you to touch me here" instead of "You touched me wrong" or "You should have touched me in other places."

The disabled partner may have to play a more passive role in sexual intercourse. Femininity or masculinity should be openly defined as different concepts in sexuality and should not depend on the physical activity of the man or woman during sexual intercourse.

Erotic zones other than the genitalia should be explored by the sexual partners, particularly when sensation is lost over the groin area. Many disabled patients have reported satisfying "mental orgasms" or sexual "highs" reminiscent of postcoital resolution and relaxation experienced prior to the injury or illness. In particular, disabled men feel less competent sexually when genital sensation becomes impaired and should be counseled appropriately.

The disabled adult with a congenital or childhood-acquired disability presents with a different set of experiences. Printed literature in this area is scarce and often based only on highly individual or anecdotal experience. The social development of the person may lag behind his or her chronologic age. Depending on the nature of the disability, the person may have little or no experience with "normal" sexual development. Many programs, however, teach principles that are often relevant to the adult with a congenital or childhood-acquired disability.

SEXUAL COUNSELING

Serious, responsible counseling of disabled people is a skill based on special experience, training, and knowledge. The pathogenesis, anatomy, physiology, and natural history of the specific disability should be understood. The counselor should feel comfortable and secure in discussing sexual matters and using sexual terms. The counselor should have the ability to deal with feelings and to help people express themselves. The counselor must suspend his or her own belief system and respect that of the disabled person.

Guidelines for working with disabled people have been suggested:*

1. Genital function alone does not make a functional relationship.

2. Urinary incontinence does not mean genital incontinence.

3. Absence of sensation does not mean absence of feelings.

4. Inability to move does not mean inability to please or be pleased.

5. The presence of deformities does not mean the absence of desire.

6. Inability to perform does not mean inability to enjoy.

7. Loss of genitals does not mean loss of sexuality.

8. Sexual dysfunction is not synonymous with personal inadequacy.

Successful counseling is based on an open, direct, sensitive, supportive relationship with the disabled person and his or her sexual partner. More effective communication between partners should be a major goal of counseling.

Planned Parenthood, mental health clinics, and rehabilitation medicine programs are often excellent resources for disabled people seeking professionally trained counselors. They may be physicians, nurses, social workers, psychologists, or other professionals familiar with physical disabilities.

REFERENCES

Becker EF: Female Sexuality Following Spinal Cord Injury. Cross L, et al (eds). Accent Special Publication, Accent on Living. Bloomington, Illinois 61701, Cheever Publishing, 1978.

Comfort A: Sexual Consequences of Disability. Philadelphia, GF Stickley, 1978.

Furlow WL: Therapy of impotence, Chap 12, pp 213–228. In Krane RJ, Siroky MB (eds): Clinical Neuro-Urology. Boston, Little, Brown, 1979.

Gregory MF: Sexual Adjustment: A Guide for the Spinal Cord Injured. Raymond C (ed). Accent Special Publication, Accent on Living. Bloomington, Illinois 61701, Cheever, 1976.

Griffith ER, Tomka MA, Timms RJ: Sexual function in spinal cord injured patients, a review. Arch Phys Med Rehabil 54:539, 1973.

Heslinga K, Schellen AM, Verkuyl A: Not Made of Stone. Springfield, Charles C Thomas, 1974.

---

*Cole TM, Cole SS: Rehabilitation of problems of sexuality in physical disability, Chap 47, p 904. In Kottke FJ, Stillwell CG, Lehmann JF (eds): Krusen's Handbook of Physical Medicine and Rehabilitation, 3rd ed. Philadelphia, Saunders, 1982.

Mooney TO, Cole TM, Chilgren RA: Sexual Options for Paraplegics and Quadriplegics. Boston, Little, Brown, 1975.

Rabin BJ: The Sensuous Wheeler: Sexual Adjustment for the Spinal Cord Injured. Multi Media Resource Center, 1525 Franklin Street, San Francisco, California, 1980.

Sha'ked A (ed): Human Sexuality and Rehabilitation Medicine, Sexual Functioning Following Spinal Cord Injury. Baltimore, Williams & Wilkins, 1981.

Task Force on Concerns of Physically Disabled Women. Towards Intimacy, Family Planning and Sexuality Concerns of Physically Disabled Women. New York, Human Sciences Press.

III

TECHNIQUES AND PROCEDURES

24

PRESCRIPTION OF THERAPY

Physical and occupational therapy may be prescribed by a physician. In many states, the law requires that a therapist possess a written prescription from a licensed physician before therapy can legally take place.

The physician should consider a prescription for therapy as a form of communication. A vague prescription will fail to convey the clinical justification for therapy. An excessively detailed prescription, however, may be inflexible and thus compromise the clinical judgment, experience, and skill of the therapist.

BASIC FORMAT

All prescriptions should contain the patient's name; specific diagnosis, condition, or problem; precautions, if any; goals of treatment; treatment duration and frequency; and the type of specific treatment with reference to the anatomic area, impaired function, and assistive devices.

Be pragmatic and keep the therapeutic goal in mind. When one is uncertain about the prescriptive content, discuss it with the therapist(s).

Temper therapy with reason. For example, avoid the prescription of four different heating modalities for each therapeutic session in the treatment of a single musculoskeletal problem.

BASIC CONTENT

Treatment Duration

Monitor progress. Recheck patients every 1–2 weeks. If therapy is efficacious, objective improvement should be observed.

Once progress levels off, consider a light home program that the physician or therapist believes has a reasonable chance of success.

For maintenance therapy based on a home program, regular rechecks by the therapist every 1–2 months are probably adequate for monitoring.

Long-term therapy prescriptions should be renewed every 3–6 months.

Therapeutic Exercise

Indicate whether exercise should be passive, assisted, or completely active. Note if the exercise should involve progressive resistance, repetitions, or a fatigue endpoint. Specify the major muscle groups and joints.

Mobility

Prescribe gait training using a prosthesis, an orthosis, or walking aids, such as canes, crutches, and walkers.

Recommend training for safe, effective wheelchair transfers, chronic sitting, and locomotion. Be specific in terms of location of activity (e.g., home, bedroom, rest room at work, or family car).

Prescribe an assessment of architectural barriers and safety at home.

Self-Care

Specify the self-care skill (dressing, undressing, grooming, hygiene, toileting). Avoid using the term "Activities of Daily Living" (ADL), which embraces many activities throughout the patient's entire day.

Prescribe the evaluation or training in the use of customized orthoses and prostheses. Prescribe specific standardized testing for hand function and visual perception.

CHECKLIST

Many departments of physical and occupational therapy prefer the use of prescriptions with checklists, as they serve to alert the physician to the range of specific therapy services. If utilized, however, checklists should be supplemented by descriptive statements from the prescribing physician. Checklists should not replace direct, critical discussion between the physician and the therapist(s).

EXAMPLE

The prescription may be written on a physician's standard prescription pad or stationery: "Dx—painful left hip secondary to DJD. Rx (1) ultrasound over 3 fields to left hip at 5–10 minutes per session, (2) isometrics for quads and gluteal muscles, (3) teach patient use of cane for right hand. Sessions 3/wk for 2 wk."

The name, address, and telephone number of the prescribing physician should appear in print on the prescription. When the physician would like to see the patient next might also appear on the prescription.

Name of Patient _____ Date _____

Diagnosis _____

Precautions _____

Goal _____

Comments:

Patient should check with me in _____weeks.

_____, MD

Name of Physician
Office address and telephone

Figure 24–1. Prototype of prescription for therapy.

25

PHYSICAL MODALITIES

MANAGEMENT OF COMMON CLINICAL PROBLEMS

Degenerative Joint Disease

Superficial heat may relieve pain secondary to muscle spasm. The deep heat of ultrasound and the immediate static stretch of the involved joint may improve joint contractures. Paraffin baths and joint range of motion may reduce the pain and stiffness of a hand with degenerative joint disease (DJD).

Rheumatoid Arthritis

In active disease, mild superficial heat may reduce pain, stiffness, and muscle spasm. Whirlpool or Hubbard tank will allow superficial heat to multiple joints.

In inactive disease, the joint contractures and stiffness of hands and feet may be managed in the same manner as chronic DJD.

Shoulder Bursitis

In the acute stage, superficial heat may relieve pain and muscle spasm. In active or chronic stages, joint contracture, calcific bursitis, and tendinitis may be treated by ultrasound and static stretch.

Contractures Secondary to Immobilization

Ultrasound to the tight joint capsule should be followed immediately by prolonged static stretch. Deep heat to contractured muscle may be best applied by low frequency microwave or shortwave diathermy. If myositis ossificans accounts for the joint contracture, an orthopedist or physiatrist should be consulted.

Joint Trauma

In acute trauma-related muscle spasms, ice treatment for 12–24 hours may effectively reduce bleeding, pain, and edema. After 48–72 hours, superficial heat may accelerate the resolution of hemorrhage and edema.

Low Back Pain

Heat or cold treatment may relieve pain and muscle spasm and thereby enhance the success of joint ranging, traction, and spinal immobilization. Ultrasound should be used cautiously in a patient recovering from a laminectomy; the intensity should be reduced. The application of ultrasound in the acute management of low back pain due to a suspected herniated disc is contraindicated. Short-wave diathermy can heat a large area of muscle and is often preferred over ultrasound. In some clinics, microwave diathermy may be suggested.

COLD MODALITIES

Cold reduces regional blood flow, collagen extensibility, and metabolic rate. Cold acutely decreases the inflammatory response and local edema. As in the application of heat, cold may reduce pain, relax muscle, and minimize spasticity.

Indications

The therapeutic effect of cold is brief, lasting from a few minutes to a few hours. Cold should be used in conjunction with other treatment to
1. Relieve pain, muscle spasm, or spasticity.
2. Reduce edema and hemorrhage in trauma and acute inflammatory reactions.
3. Facilitate muscle contraction in some forms of neurogenic weakness.

Contraindications

Cold is contraindicated in the presence of ischemia or impaired local tissue circulation. Patients with cold sensitivity, such as in Raynaud's syndrome, cryoglobulinemia, paroxysmal cold hemoglobinuria, and marked cold pressor response, should avoid cold treatment.

Equipment

The equipment is simple: packs filled with crushed ice, frozen gel packs, or ice water baths. As the primary coolant melts, it should be replaced promptly.

Prescription

For superficial tissues, immersion in ice water for 10–30 minutes is probably sufficient. For deeper tissues, 60 minutes or more is necessary. The exchange of cold across the insulating layer acts to retard warming of the cooled deeper tissue. Ice massage does not cool superficial or deep tissues and is used to facilitate muscle retraining and control. The application of cold for spasticity or neuromuscular facilitation should be done by a trained physical or occupational therapist. For the physician, cold is most useful in the treatment of edema, bleeding, and pain due to local tissue trauma.

HYDROTHERAPY

Hydrotherapy is the external use of water in the treatment of diseases. There are three therapeutic modalities of hydrotherapy: chemicals with antiseptic iodine solution, mechanical agitation, and superficial heat.

Equipment

The whirlpool tub is a small tank capable of allowing immersion of a limb or two at a time. The Hubbard tank is large and permits the total immersion of limbs or the body itself up to the neck. The tanks are costly to procure and to operate.

A swimming pool warmed to 30.0–32.2°C (86–90°F) can provide the opportunity for supervised therapeutic exercises that are more difficult for the disabled person to complete without the buoyancy of deep water. In recreation, **adaptive aquatics** is very popular.

A Water Pik is a device effective in the debridement of decubiti and other necrotic wounds. In other situations, a whirlpool, Hubbard tank, or deep bathtub equipped with an agitator may be excellent for thorough, vigorous hydrotherapy of a large necrotic wound.

Prescription

The temperature settings are as follows:

1. Whirlpool tub: 37.8–38.9°C (100–102°F) for legs and 37.8–40.6°C (100–105°F) for upper extremities. With selective limb immersion, temperatures up to 43.3–46.0°C (110–115°F) have been applied. The anatomic site may be submerged for 20–30 minutes b.i.d.

2. Hubbard tank: 36.7–37.2°C (98–99°F) for mild heating and 37.8–38.3°C (100–101°F) for vigorous heating involving immersion of the body. For the elderly or patients with marginal cardiovascular function, vital signs should be monitored and the patient closely supervised when the total body is immersed and the temperatures are high. They should not exceed 38.9–39.4°C (102–103°F).

3. Swimming pool: 30.0–32.2°C (86–90°F) for therapeutic exercises in patients with arthritis or spasticity.

4. Fine water jet stream: tepid or room temperature water.

Precautions

Patients with cardiovascular impairment should be monitored closely in a heated Hubbard tank. Core body temperature, pulse rate, and cardiovascular demands may rise significantly. Heart failure or arrhythmia may be precipitated. High-risk patients should not be left unattended.

Equipment should be meticulously scrubbed with antiseptic solution. Health standards should be met without fail. Most of this equipment is used in hospital or clinic settings and is subject to strict operational policies and procedures.

The physician's prescription should contain information on any precaution relevant to the patient's treatment. Congestive heart failure, osteoporosis, seizures, and other pertinent data should appear. For some patients, the therapist should be requested to monitor blood pressure, pulse rate, respiratory rate, and mental status. The physician may wish to inquire about the level of water safety supervision and emergency backup.

To avoid accidental scalding burns, home gas or electric heaters should have their thermostats set at 49.0–52.0°C (120–125°F) or lower. Full-thickness burns can take place in 10–20 minutes. Disabled people are more prone to this preventable injury.

HEAT MODALITIES

Heat increases regional blood flow, collagen extensibility, and metabolic rate. Heat acutely increases the inflammatory response and edema of tissue. As it raises the pain threshold, pain is thereby reduced. Heat relaxes muscle and reduces spasticity.

General Indications

The therapeutic effect of heat is brief, lasting from a few minutes to a few hours. It should be used in conjunction with other treatment.

Heat can relieve pain, muscle spasms, or spasticity. Used in conjunction with static stretch, heat may reduce contractures. Heat may facilitate the resolution of inflammatory edema and exudate, as well as the reduction of joint stiffness.

Contraindications

Avoid heat as a treatment in patients with a hemorrhagic diathesis (for example, a hemophiliac joint with active bleeding); acute trauma, including sprained joints and bruises; malignancies, particularly involving the tissue receiving the heat; ischemic tissue;

and active inflammatory conditions, such as acute, active rheumatoid arthritis. Some deep-heating modalities may be contraindicated in the presence of a metal prosthesis, such as a hip joint implant. The patient in a coma or with paralysis, insensate skin, or full debilitation is at great risk for thermal injury.

Superficial and Deep Heat

Superficial heat involves the skin and subcutaneous layers. Deep heat involves muscle and joint capsule. If properly applied, deep heat does not generally heat superficial tissue.

The therapeutic effect of heat is attained when the target tissue receives the greatest concentration of heat. The therapeutic effect of heat may occur whether the source is moist, dry, or from a lamp. Unfortunately, there is no precise dosimetry in heat therapy. The effectiveness, ease of application, precautions, and adverse effects may differ considerably among the different sources.

Types of Heat Sources

Superficial heat: heating lamp, electric heating pad, hot water bottle, hot packs, and paraffin bath. **Deep heat:** ultrasound, shortwave, and microwave.

Superficial Heat

Application for 20–30 minutes b.i.d. is usually sufficient and produces no further benefit beyond that treatment frequency. Because the involved body surface may be covered by the heating source itself, thermal burns can occur easily. **Impaired sensation or circulation may predispose the skin to severe burns.**

Heat Lamps *(ordinary light bulb, tungsten filament lamp, carbon tungsten lamp, mercury vapor lamp)*

Heat lamps have very limited therapeutic indication and are prescribed most often to dry, moist, and weeping skin lesions. Their use is simple and they may be used at home.

Prescription: 100- to 150-watt bulb, 35–75 cm from the skin. Heat for 20–30 minutes b.i.d. Concentrate the heat by shaping the shiny side of aluminum foil half around the bulb or inside the lamp reflector.

Precautions: Advise the patient to **stabilize the lamp securely** to prevent it from falling on the skin. Recommend that the patient or attendant touch and look at the site of heating, particularly when an anesthetic lesion is being treated.

Electric Heating Pad

Mild ankle sprain and other mild musculoskeletal trauma may be helped by an electric heating pad. Pain may be relieved and local circulation enhanced. It is simple and may be used at home. The need for steady heat, however, predisposes the patient to inadvertent burns, particularly when the patient lies on the heating pad.

Place the part of the body **under,** not on, the heating pad for 20–30 minutes every 4–12 hours. Avoid high settings on the thermostat and discourage the patient from lying on the pad.

Hot Water Bottle

Its clinical indications are similar to those of the electric heating pad. Because water cools rapidly in such a container, the heat dissipates quickly. Burns, however, may still occur from a hot bottle or from scalding water leaking from the bottle.

Water may be heated to 65.6°C (150°F), which is often the thermal limit for the glass container. Three to six bath towels are placed **between** the skin and the bottle. It is applied for 20–30 minutes b.i.d. The body part is placed **under** the bottle and towels. Single layers may be removed as the temperature of the bottle cools.

Precaution: Do **not** place the bottle in direct contact with the skin unless the bottle is tolerable to touch.

Hot Towel

Its indications are similar to those of the electric heating pad. It has extremely limited application and in most cases is not recommended. The towel is drenched in hot water and excess water is wrung out of it. The therapeutic heating time is only 5 minutes because of rapid dissipation of heat. Thus, when the towel becomes cool enough to handle comfortably, the heating effect will probably be subtherapeutic.

Contrast Bath

The immersion of arthritic fingers, hands, feet, and ankles into alternating baths of hot and cold water produces hyperemia in stiff, painful joints and can reduce symptoms effectively. The temperature is 40.6–43.3°C (105–110°F) for the hot water and 15.0°–20.0°C (59–68°F) for the cold water.

The protocol begins with a 10-minute hot immersion of the involved joints, followed by 1 minute of cold immersion. The patient returns to the hot water for 4 minutes, then to the cold water for 1 minute. This 4:1 bathing continues for the balance of a 30-minute treatment session.

Hydrocollator Packs

These packs are silicate gel enveloped by canvas. Their application is similar to that of the electric heating pad. Most therapists will use hydrocollator packs when a prescription requests "hot packs." These durable packs do not require wringing out of hot, excess water. They may be utilized at home.

The most commonly used packs measure 50 × 50 cm and thus cover a relatively small area, such as the low back or ankle. Pack temperatures reach 71.1–79.4°C (160–175°F).

Several bath towels or terry cloths should be **interposed** between the hydrocollator pack and the skin. The position of the body should be **under** the pack. The application takes 20–30 minutes. b.i.d. For the perineum, a small hydrocollator pack (about half the average size) may be ordered. The therapist or an attendant should inspect the skin and touch the affected skin periodically during treatment to avoid burn or subtherapeutic application.

Sample instructions to the patient for home application:

Hydrocollator steam packs can be purchased at surgical supply houses and some drug stores. Place packs in a pan at least 2 in. (5 cm) deep and fill with water. Soak packs overnight. Heat on stove until water just starts to boil. Remove pack from the pan and wrap it with 8–10 thicknesses of bath towels. Place it over the area to be treated. If the pack is **too cold**, remove some of the towels until the heat is barely comfortable. If the pack is **too hot**, add another layer of towel until it is barely comfortable. Packs should be left on the body part for 20–30 minutes but should remain warm during this time. After treatment, place packs back in water until the next treatment. When the pack is to be used no longer, allow it to dry for several days and the pack will shrink up for storage. This pack can be used over and over again for an indefinite period of time.

Paraffin Bath

Paraffin baths are usually applied for hand or foot problems, particularly subacute or chronic arthritis, when pain and restricted joint range of motion require improvement.

A bath can cover the entire surface of the hand or foot. The heat is retained for a full 30 minutes. The paraffin leaves the skin soft and moist. Because of its unique penetration in the hands and feet, paraffin heat may effectively reach chronically stiff joints in rheumatoid arthritis. New skin and scar tissue do not tolerate intense paraffin heating.

The dipping technique may be selected to apply paraffin from a 52.2–59.4°C (126–130°F) bath (6:1 **paraffin to mineral oil**) 20–30 minutes b.i.d.–t.i.d. Follow the heat treatment with active to passive range of motion to the involved joints.

Precaution: Use a thermometer to check the bath temperature at regular intervals. In rheumatoid arthritis, apply the paraffin heat to **only chronic**, quiescent joints of the hand and possibly feet. Avoid heating acutely inflamed joints. Utilize the proper equipment to heat the paraffin and mineral oil. A double boiler or commercial paraffin heaters are available at commercial medical supply houses.

Sample instruction to the patient for home treatment:

Equipment: double boiler (6-quart or greater capacity); thermometer, measuring up to at least 57.2°C (135°F); paper towel, brown wrapping paper or wax paper sufficient to cover the hands or feet; bath towel or bath blanket.

Ingredients: mineral oil, 340 g or 12 oz.; paraffin, 450 g or 1 lb; tap water to fill the lower half of the double boiler.

Fill the lower half of the double boiler with water to avoid burning the paraffin. Add paraffin and mineral oil in a 6:1 ratio (6 parts of paraffin to every 1 part of mineral oil). Heat the mixture to 52.2–54.4°C (126–130°F).

Dip the hand(s) or feet into the paraffin bath up to the wrist or ankle quickly in and out. Allow the paraffin to solidify. Redip. Repeat this process 8–10 times, until a thick "glove" for the hand or "boot" for the foot is formed.

Wrap the glove with paper, then a bath towel or blanket for 20–30 minutes. Remove the paraffin by slipping a finger under the upper edge of the glove or boot. Peel paraffin off.

The paraffin dip may be performed twice a day. Your physician and therapist may prescribe stretch exercises for your joints immediately following the paraffin treatment.

Deep Heat

Ultrasound

Ultrasound may be used to treat the contracture of the periarticular soft tissue following prolonged immobilization, rheumatic inflammation, DJD, and trauma.

Ultrasound may be of value in the treatment of reflex sympathetic dystrophy (shoulder-hand syndrome), postherpetic pain, tennis elbow, painful neuroma in amputated limbs, and contractured joints.

Ultrasound is the only heat modality that will affect the periarticular joint structures well. Unlike short-wave and microwave diathermy, ultrasound can be applied over joints with metallic prostheses or implants.

Ultrasound can produce deep burns quickly. Its therapeutic effect is best achieved when the tissue is heated just short of burning. Ultrasound requires meticulous attention to proper technique of application and can be easily applied incorrectly. Ultrasound does not heat the skin and subcutaneous layers and so, because of the absence of this warning stimulus, it should be applied by a trained **physical or occupational therapist.** If a contractured joint is receiving ultrasound, the joint should be stretched during or immediately after ultrasound treatment.

Ultrasound should **not** be applied around the eyes, over a pregnant uterus, or over acutely inflamed joints or tissue. Because ultrasound may promote tissue swelling, lumbar disc herniation and secondary nerve root compression may be aggravated by ultrasound therapy.

Short-wave and Microwave Diathermy

These two modalities are highly specialized in their application. Short-wave diathermy may cover a large area, such as the back, shoulder, and hip, as well as parts of the upper and lower extremities. It should **not** be applied to a patient with a cardiac pacemaker. Metallic prosthetic implants, metal-containing intra-uterine devices, contact lenses, and metal overlying skin (e.g., watches, jewelry, buckles) should be avoided. The beads of per-spiration should be absorbed by a terry cloth over the patient's skin. Short-wave diathermy may increase menstrual hemorrhage and, until proven safe, should not be administered to pregnant women or over epiphyseal growth centers in children. The patient should lie on a wooden treatment table or chair.

The use of short-wave or microwave diathermy requires continual supervision by an experienced physical or occupational therapist. The use of equipment should be restricted to a therapy clinic and is **inappropriate for routine "office" use.**

Place of Treatment

When a patient and family are reliable, responsible, and intelli-gent, superficial heat modalities may be recommended for home use. Deep heat modalities, however, involve electrical equipment, specialized supervision, and potentially dangerous complications. They are used almost exclusively in hospital or clinic settings and applied by physical or occupational therapists.

Heat therapy alone is rarely sufficient. Static stretch of contrac-tured joints or muscles, strengthening of muscle groups, and compliant use of prescribed medication, for example, may be equally important to the improvement of the patient.

The prescription and application of heat, superficial or deep, should not be regarded as innocuous therapy by patient, physician, or therapist. Serious thermal burns, for example, have resulted from injudicious behavior, improper technique, abuse, faulty equipment, and inadequate supervision. Similar causes have re-sulted in subtherapeutic doses of heat and costly sessions with negative therapeutic value.

REFERENCES

Lehmann JF (ed): Therapeutic Heat and Cold, 3rd ed. Baltimore, Williams & Wilkins, 1982.

Lehmann JF, DeLateur BJ: Diathermy and superficial heat and cold therapy, Chap 13, pp 275–350. In Kottke FJ, Stillwell GK, Lehmann JF (eds): Krusen's Handbook of Physical Medicine and Rehabilitation, 3rd ed. Philadelphia, Saun-ders, 1982.

Licht S (ed): Medical Hydrology. New Haven, Elizabeth Licht, 1963.

26

MASSAGE

Massage is the manipulation of soft tissues with the hands to produce a therapeutic effect. Massage may be augmented by powder, oil, or water. Its effect may last for 20–60 minutes. The frequency of massage varies from b.i.d. to weekly.

Massage appears to have physiologic effects. Light stroking of the skin produces a mild capillary constriction, or a white reaction. Heavy stroking and friction produce a triple response of red reaction, wheal, and flare. Greater capillary flow and arteriolar dilatation occur. Massage may increase local venous circulation, lymph drainage in an extremity, and relaxation of muscle. Localized adhesions, fibrous scars, and trigger points may be stretched or disrupted by massage. As in other forms of "hands on" therapy, the psychologic effect of massage is important.

TYPES OF MASSAGE

Effleurage, or stroking, is performed superficially or deeply in a distal to proximal direction. Stroking serves to improve local circulation, lymph drainage, and relaxation.

Petrissage, or compression, consists of kneading, squeezing, skin rolling, and muscle compression. Used over large areas, kneading may create better relaxation, improve local circulation, and reduce muscle tightness.

Friction, a form of petrissage, is performed in a circular or rolling manner over small areas of tendon, muscle, or ligament. Such massage reduces adhesions following sprains, strains, muscle pulls, or tendinitis. It may be used at musculotendinous junctions that have been injured and are painful.

Tapotement, or percussion, involves hacking, clapping, beating, or pounding to improve blood flow, sensory stimulation, and pulmonary drainage.

Ice massage consists of rubbing ice over the skin to facilitate muscle re-education. Cooler temperatures in the underlying tissue, however, require large ice chip packs or ice-water immersion.

PRECAUTIONS

Cutaneous inflammation (infectious and noninfectious), burns, underlying malignant masses, clotting disorders, fractures, and thrombophlebitis are contraindications to massage.

THERAPEUTIC CONSIDERATIONS

It is difficult to evaluate massage as a therapy. The method, however, has survived centuries and is applied widely in nonmedical settings. Massage is unquestionably efficacious in individuals with certain kinds of soft tissue ailments. Practitioners of massage do not pretend that it is the panacea for all bodily "aches and pains" or that it is a substitute for other well-established forms of medical or surgical treatment.

REFERENCES

Cyriax J: Deep massage. Physiotherapy 63:60, 1977.
Ebner M: Connective tissue massage. Physiotherapy 64:208, 1978.
Rogoff JB (ed): Manipulation, Traction and Massage, 2nd ed. Baltimore, Williams & Wilkins, 1980.
Wood EC, Becker PD: Beard's Massage, 3rd ed. Philadelphia, Saunders, 1981.

27

MANIPULATION

Manipulation involves passive movement of a joint for therapeutic purposes. To many practitioners, the short, rapid, forceful movement of small excursion at or near the ends of joint range constitutes manipulation.

Manipulation of peripheral joints increases joint range by stretching tight ligaments and, in some instances, breaking adhesions. Manipulation may realign intrasynovial structures, such as displaced meniscus.

Spine manipulation appears to work well in some patients for reasons that are most often unclear. The extruded disc material may be repositioned. Large diameter sensory nerves may be excited, thus closing the "pain gate." Muscle relaxation may be achieved by the stretch of small back rotator muscles. The high "tone" caused by the sympathetic nervous system may be reduced in the spinal segment. Stretch of the interspinal and capsular ligaments or adhesions may improve joint range. "Locked facets" and entrapped nerve fibers may be released by manipulation. These mechanisms have been advanced as explanations for the effect of manipulation.

TYPES OF MANIPULATION

Peripheral manipulation consists of anterior-posterior glide, lateral glide, distraction, tilt (flexion and extension), and rotation.

Spinal manipulation involves rotation, anterior-posterior glide, tilt (lateral flexion, forward flexion, and extension), and distraction in combination with any of the above.

Manipulative movements involve the standard range of motion that uses slow pressure throughout the full arch of joint range. Mobilization entails slow, oscillating movements at the ends of joint range. Manipulation requires rapid, short amplitude movements at the ends of joint range.

THERAPEUTIC CONSIDERATION

Clinical Indications

A. Loss of joint range of motion in a peripheral limb, secondary to immobilization due to trauma or capsular inflammation.

B. Mildly or partially ruptured disc. Extreme caution should be used. The practitioner must be alert to dural or root signs of compression. Distraction should be used concomitantly.

C. Tight spinal segment. Manipulation or stretch may aggravate the symptoms if the adjoining loose segment is painful on movement.

D. Placebo effect. Other forms of treatment should be used if manipulation is being employed only for its "hands-on" placebo effect.

Precautions or Contraindications

Manipulation may increase joint fluid or overstretch inflamed ligaments in inflammatory conditions. For joint effusions, the technique of mobilization, not manipulation, should be initially tried. In degenerative joint disease (DJD) of the spine, manipulation may exacerbate pain symptoms and produce an effusion. Manipulation should be avoided in moderate to severe nerve root impingement. Manipulation of the cervical spine may precipitate an embolic or thrombotic stroke in patients over age 55 with a history of athcrosclerotic disease. A joint with increased laxity from a ligamentous rupture should not be manipulated.

Practitioners

The techniques of manipulation have been incorporated into the practice of orthopedic surgeons, physiatrists, physical therapists, and occupational therapists. However, manipulation as the major or only form of treatment for all painful syndromes of soft tissue cannot be scientifically justified.

REFERENCES

Cyriax JH: Treatment by manipulation, massage and injection. In Textbook of Orthopedic Medicine, Vol 2. Baltimore, Williams & Wilkins, 1977.
Maitland GD: Vertebral Manipulation, 4th ed. Boston, Butterworths, 1977.
Rogoff JB (ed): Manipulation, Traction and Massage, 2 ed. Baltimore, Williams & Wilkins, 1980.

28

BIOFEEDBACK

Biofeedback refers to any process that monitors a physiologic response in a patient and provides specific information concerning concurrent biologic changes. The information is presented in such a way that the patient can learn to self-regulate the physiologic function being monitored.

Biofeedback assumes that for each emotional or mental change there exists a corresponding physiologic change. Conversely, for each physiologic change, there exists a corresponding emotional or mental change.

EQUIPMENT

The equipment is designed to sample specific physiologic activity rapidly and accurately. There are five major types of biofeedback equipment. Electromyographic equipment monitors muscle; thermal, peripheral vasculature; cardiovascular, heart rate and blood pressure; electroencephalographic, brain waves; and electrodermal, skin impedance.

CLINICAL INDICATIONS

Pain Control

Tension headache, neck pain, shoulder pain, upper back pain, lower back pain, and myofascial pain in the absence of nerve damage, such as temporal mandibular joint pain, bruxism, and generalized pain from muscle tension, are common clinical conditions. Electromyographic equipment is used. Biofeedback may be insufficient when muscle spasm or tension is absent in the area of "pain," when other parts of the body do not show any evidence of muscle spasm or tension, or when the patient has a chronic history of pain that is refractory to conventional medical management.

Chronic pain may require an evaluation and referral to experienced physicians or psychologists.

Neuromuscular Re-Education

This applies to lower extremity spasms in incomplete spinal cord injury, lower extremity spasticity following cerebrovascular accident, lower extremity incoordination in cerebral palsy and cerebrovascular accident, hand incoordination following cerebrovascular accident and head trauma, and facial tics related to Bell's palsy.

The equipment is electromyographic. Biofeedback augments basic rehabilitative treatment.

Stress Management

Hypertension, free-floating anxiety, phobias, and insomnia are examples of clinical conditions. Electromyographic equipment is used. Stress is thought to be aggravated or caused by muscle tension. Biofeedback is used to teach a patient to relax.

Temperature-Associated Conditions

Classic migraine headache, idiopathic Raynaud's phenomenon, peripheral vascular disease, and hypertension are specific conditions. The equipment utilizes thermal monitoring and involves placement of sensitive thermistors over peripheral skin, such as the fingertips or forehead. Changes as small as 0.1–.01°F can be detected by this method.

An increase in peripheral temperature suggests a relaxation of the sympathetic nervous system. Patients, however, usually find electromyographic feedback easier to learn in the management of stress. For any stress-related disorder, the electromyographic method should be tried first.

Hypertension

The patient learns how to control systolic and diastolic blood pressures. A reduction in medication may follow. The equipment utilizes a cannula transducer implanted in a major artery or an occluding cuff and stethoscope. An experienced practitioner should supervise the biofeedback therapy initially.

Brain Dysfunction

Seizures, chronic pain, hyperactivity, anxiety, and insomnia are specific conditions that have been treated with electroencephalographic biofeedback. The interest in brain wave feedback stemmed from the observation that yoga meditators exhibit pain and body physiology control and produce significant increases in the proportion of alpha wave activity. Subjects learned to alter their brain wave patterns significantly.

Clinical application is very limited because of the expensive equipment, specialized monitoring, and preliminary studies based on only a few patients.

Other Conditions

Biofeedback practitioners have reported limited success in the following areas: speech disorders, such as stuttering, subvocalization, and voice quality deficits; tinnitus; asthma; gastrointestinal disorders, such as functional diarrhea, encopresis, neurogenic fecal incontinence, urinary retention, urinary incontinence, and ulcerative colitis; and sexual dysfunction, such as erectile failure and orgasmic dysfunction.

MANAGEMENT

The practitioner of biofeedback should possess the training, knowledge, and clinical judgment necessary to evaluate and treat patients appropriately, properly, and effectively.

Biofeedback is not a substitute for conventional medical or surgical treatment. In most settings, biofeedback is noninvasive. For patients with physical disabilities, biofeedback may be selectively effective in the management of anxiety, muscle spasm, chronic pain, and neuromuscular re-education.

REFERENCES

Basmajian J (ed): Biofeedback, Principles and Practice for Clinicians. Baltimore, Williams & Wilkins, 1979.
Biofeedback Society of America, 4301 Owens Street, Wheat Ridge, Colorado 80033. A professional directory is published.

29

TRANSCUTANEOUS ELECTRICAL NERVE STIMULATION

Transcutaneous electrical nerve stimulation (TENS or TNS) is a battery-powered device that electrostimulates overlying skin for pain relief. The Gate Control Theory (Melzak and Wall) suggests that selective stimulation of cutaneous sensory fibers may inhibit the perception of pain.

CLINICAL INDICATIONS

In chronic pain conditions, TENS may symptomatically relieve pain. It may be used concurrently with physical or occupational therapy. It is not clearly known which patient is the optimal candidate. Results have varied between success and failure.

In acute pain, relatively good success has been found in patients who experience postoperative pain from abdominal surgery, thoracic surgery, and laminectomies. The use of TENS in acute back pain, arthritis, and bursitis is less clearly established.

The only relative contraindication is a moderate to severe reaction to the tape, electrical stimuli, or conducting medium. A change in tape or electrode gel usually resolves the adverse effect.

Absolute contraindications include the following: use over cardiac pacemakers, carotid sinus, pregnant uterus, phrenic nerve pacers, or insulin pump, or in the presence of electronic life support mechanisms.

EQUIPMENT

Different TENS units produce different electrical waveforms. The most effective waveform, however, has not been determined. Empirically, the waveform may be adjusted in amplitude, frequency, and duration to relieve pain maximally for an individual patient.

Several units should be tried on a patient to determine the optimal waveform. Each unit should have variable current amplitude, pulse width, and pulse rate.

In the adjustment of a TENS unit, the sensory fiber stimulation occurs optimally when high-frequency, short-duration electrical impulses are applied at an adequate amplitude. Pulse rate should be preset at 70–150 pulses per second (pps). Pulse width should be less than 130 microseconds (μsec). The amplitude should be set at a comfortable level of intensity.

The patient may adjust the intensity of current, but the physician or therapist should adjust the pulse rate and width.

Empirically, the optimal location for electrode placement is determined by the physician or therapist. The sites may be trigger points, acupuncture points, discrete areas of greatest pain, along peripheral nerves, and along dermatomes or spinal segmental levels that cross the area of pain.

Continuous application may produce skin irritation. Although the pattern of use varies from individual to individual, many patients discover a carry-over effect, which reduces the use of the TENS on a continuous basis.

Initially, the TENS unit is used continuously until the pain is brought under control. After 3–7 days of continuous use, the patient is encouraged to turn the TENS off periodically. The off-time is increased as long as pain control is maintained.

MANAGEMENT

Short training courses are available for physicians interested in learning, applying, and supervising the use of TENS units. In the event the physician chooses to consult a trained, experienced physical or occupational therapist in TENS intervention, the following **guidelines** should be considered: Set up an initial trial period of 1 month. If significant relief of pain occurs during the first 3–5 days, continue the rest of the month. If the patient derives significant benefit during this trial period, it is likely that TENS will have a long-term benefit.

The patient should understand the principles of TENS intervention. The electrodes should be placed properly and adeptly. Rent a TENS unit until it is clearly established that it will have long-term value. Urge the patient to comply with other aspects of the overall management program.

REFERENCES

Melzak R, Wall P: Pain mechanisms, a new theory. Science *150*:971, 1965.
Symposium of TENS use. Phys Ther *58*:1443, 1978.

30

PERIPHERAL NERVE BLOCKS

The selective injection of anesthetic or neurolytic material around a peripheral nerve can effectively paralyze those muscles innervated by the nerve. The nerve may be blocked anywhere along its trunk or at the point proximal to or near the terminal innervation within the muscle, which has been referred to as **intramuscular neurolysis** or motor point block.

CLINICAL INDICATIONS

Diagnostic. The temporary anesthetic block to a peripheral nerve may simulate or approximate the clinical outcome of a proposed tenotomy or neurectomy. For example, anesthetic block of the obturator nerve can produce major paralysis of the hip adductors.

Joint range may be more accurately measured by passive movement and goniometry when a tight, spastic muscle is difficult to control or when it is not clear whether the tightness is dynamic or fixed.

A temporary block may allow assessment of potential muscle imbalance or voluntary motor control in a patient with problems in spasticity.

Therapeutic. When a spastic muscle group interferes with mobility or self-care, a block should be considered. The spastic muscle can predispose a joint to harmful contractures and can create a muscle imbalance about a joint. Patients with spinal cord injury, cerebrovascular accident, traumatic brain injury, or cerebral palsy commonly have spastic muscles, which may be managed by blocks.

EQUIPMENT

A pulse generator is an electrostimulator, capable of square wave, direct current impulses. The equipment can have a current range of 0–10 milliamperes (ma), a pulse duration range of 0.1–0.5 millisecond (msec), and a frequency range of 1–2 per second.

The cathode is a hollow, Teflon-coated 22- to 24-gauge "motor point" needle, 2–5 in. (5.0–12.5 cm) in length. Its tip is beveled, exposed metal. The needle base may be clipped to an insulated wire that leads to the pulse generator. The indifferent electrode may be a gauze foam pad, which is soaked with water or saline and placed under the body part being treated.

BLOCKING AGENTS

Short-acting lidocaine 1% may be mixed with long-acting bupivacaine (0.25% or 0.50%) or chloroprocaine 2% to bring about prompt and prolonged effect of up to 2–6 hours. Thus, the patient, family, therapist, or nurse will have the opportunity to observe and work with the patient for specific functional activities, such as walking, sitting, or self care.

> **Extreme caution** should be used when employing large volumes of anesthetic. The procedure is less blind if the pulse generator is utilized to localize the peripheral nerve precisely. Volumes less than 1–2 ml may be injected. Precaution is taken to avoid intravascular injection. "Blind" injections of large volumes of any of the anesthetic agents are potentially dangerous and should be performed by an experienced physician with proper standby emergency resources.

Phenol 5% is preferred by some physicians as an effective neurolytic agent. Other alcohol solutions have also been recommended. Clear clinical benefits usually range between 3 and 9 months. The chemical lysis of mixed sensory-motor nerves may produce excellent results in paralyzing the innervated muscles. Causalgia, however, has been reported. Apparently, afferent sensory nerve fibers become chemically irritated and cause dysesthetic pain, paresthesia, or hyperesthesia. For this reason, mixed nerves are seldom blocked with phenol.

COMMONLY BLOCKED PERIPHERAL NERVES

In the **upper extremity**, the median, musculocutaneous, and ulnar nerves have been blocked temporarily. Intramuscular neurolysis with phenol has been performed on such muscles as the biceps, brachialis, wrist flexor (flexor carpi ulnaris or radialis), flexor digitorum, flexor pollicis, adductor pollicis, and pronator teres.

In the **lower extremity**, the obturator, femoral, posterior tibial, common peroneal, and popliteal nerves have been blocked temporarily. Neurolysis of the obturator nerve, however, has not produced causalgia and can be an effective method of reducing hip adductor spasticity. Intramuscular neurolysis with phenol has been performed on the gastrocnemius, soleus, tibialis posterior, hamstring, adductors, tensor fascia lata, and gluteus maximus.

ADVERSE EFFECTS

The search for the "motor points" within muscle may be tedious, painful, and traumatic. Patients may complain of muscular discomfort for 1–2 weeks following the procedure. Most patients do not need analgesics. Vigorous passive range of motion is usually discouraged for 4–7 days to avoid tears.

The electrostimulation is uncomfortable and usually occurs when higher current is used to locate the general territory of the "motor point." For most of the procedure, however, the current is tolerated well.

Pain, paresthesia, dysesthesia, or hyperesthesia may occur in 10–15% of patients in whom major mixed peripheral nerves have been blocked by a neurolytic agent, such as phenol or ethanol. The incidence increases to 15–20% in repeat peripheral nerve blocks. There is no symptomatic cure. Analgesics, tranquilizers, and muscle relaxants do not relieve the symptoms, which abate spontaneously within 1–2 months.

The block may allow the antagonist muscle group to create an imbalance about the joint in a direction opposite that of the blocked agonist muscle group.

The block may take away the pattern of extension, flexion, abduction, or adduction that the patient has come to rely on for standing, pivot transfers, walking, and reaching.

A temporary loss of balance or motor control may occur dramatically after a block and create a sense of insecurity or instability in the patient.

These adverse effects may be obviated by judicious selection of candidates for phenol or neurolytic blocks. Occasionally, an initial injection of a temporary block (e.g., lidocaine and bupivacaine) is indicated. If the anesthetic block is successful, the physician can schedule a more permanent block within a few days.

MANAGEMENT

The effect of phenol is not permanent. Although it can be repeated, scar tissue makes each subsequent block more difficult to perform rapidly. Thus, **neurolytic blocks should always complement other treatment,** such as physical or occupational therapy. During their period of greatest effect, effort should be made to teach the patient selective motor control, to increase joint range of motion, and to improve specific functional activities.

In adults, general anesthesia may be required for a patient to tolerate the procedure. The vast majority of patients, however, tolerate the procedure well. Some physicians recommend general anesthesia for children undergoing blocks.

REFERENCES

Easton JKM, Turkyilmax O, Halpern D: Intramuscular neurolysis for spasticity in children. Arch Phys Med Rehabil 60:155, 1979.

Khalili AA, Betts, HB: Management of Spasticity with Phenol Nerve Block. Chicago, Rehabilitation Institute of Chicago, 1970.

Moore DC: Regional Block, 4th ed. Springfield Ill., Charles C Thomas, 1969.

31

ELECTRODIAGNOSIS

Electrodiagnosis involves the electrophysiologic measurement of nerve and muscle function by **electromyography** (EMG) or **nerve conduction velocities** (NCVs). EMG involves a needle electrode, which is used to probe muscle for normal or abnormal electrical potentials during muscle relaxation or contraction. Nerve conduction study measures the velocity with which motor or sensory fibers can conduct an electrical impulse.

INDICATIONS

Electrodiagnosis may be used to evaluate the integrity of the **primary motor unit**, which includes the anterior horn cell, nerve root, peripheral nerve, neuromuscular junction, and the innervated muscle fibers.

A study may confirm a clinical diagnosis, localize the site of the dysfunction, establish the completeness of the dysfunction, differentiate between chronic and acute dysfunction, and rule out malingering symptoms.

Electrodiagnostic evaluation may be warranted in the following conditions:

A. **Anterior horn cell:** amyotrophic lateral sclerosis, poliomyelitis, spinal muscular atrophy, syringomyelia.

B. **Nerve root:** radiculopathy secondary to a herniated intervertebral disc or narrow foramina, radiculitis.

C. **Peripheral nerve:** polyneuropathy associated with diabetes mellitus, uremia, alcoholism, heavy metal ingestion, heredity (e.g., Charcot-Marie-Tooth disease), trauma, Guillain-Barré polyradiculoneuritis.

Entrapment of peripheral nerves including median, radial, ulnar, suprascapular, C7–T1 (thoracic outlet syndrome), femoral, sciatic, lateral femoral cutaneous, peroneal, and tibial nerves.

Brachial, lumbar, or sacral plexus injury, compression, or inflammation.

D. **Neuromuscular junction:** myasthenia gravis, botulism, Eaton-Lambert syndrome.

E. **Muscle:** myopathy, dystrophy, myositis.

EQUIPMENT

Many instrument companies manufacture modular equipment for electrodiagnostic studies. All equipment capable of EMG or

NCV studies have an amplifier, cathode ray tube (CRT) or oscilloscope, audio-speaker, and electrostimulator. In EMG, the electrodes are needles 23–27 gauge in diameter and metal discs 1.0–2.5 cm round. In nerve conduction studies, the stimulator may have metal prongs or soft pads as cathodes and anodes. Electrode gel or saline is used to reduce skin impedance.

Over the past 5 years, modular equipment has been expanded to perform **visual, auditory,** and **somesthetic evoked potentials** in addition to the conventional EMG and peripheral sensory or motor nerve conduction studies.

Electromyography

In most routine evaluations, an active needle electrode is inserted into the belly of the sampled muscle. A reference surface disc electrode is taped to the skin nearby. A ground, which is usually a large metal disc taped to the skin, acts as a "sink" for stray or background electrical "noise." A saline-soaked cloth cuff is sometimes preferred as the ground. The needle picks up activity that is translated directly into waveforms appearing on the CRT and into audio signals from a speaker. Some EMG machines can produce a hard copy of the oscilloscopic activity.

Nerve Conduction Velocity

In most routine studies, a small active electrode disc is taped over the belly of the muscle, which is innervated by the peripheral nerve under evaluation. A similar reference disc is taped distal to the active electrode. A ground is taped between the site of stimulation and the active electrode. The stimulator is a plastic handle that holds the cathode and anode. It is placed firmly over the skin and held until the electrostimulation is completed. For sensory stimulation of the hands, elastic conductive ring electrodes may be used.

Normal values of a few commonly obtained nerve conduction velocities are as follows:

Median nerve
  Wrist to thenar muscle latency (time) 3.7 ± 0.3 msec
  Elbow to wrist NCV 57 ± 5 m/sec
Ulnar nerve
  Wrist to hypothenar mucle latency 3.2 ± 0.5 msec
  Below elbow to wrist NCV 59 ± 5 m/sec
Peroneal nerve
  Ankle to m. extensor digitorum brevis 4.5 ± 0.8 msec
    latency
  Below fibular head to ankle NCV 52 ± 4 m/sec
Tibial nerve
  Medial malleolus to plantar muscles $3.4–3.9 \pm .5$ msec
    latencies

Knee to anckle NCV	55 ± 8 m/sec
Sensory nerve fibers	
Median, wrist to digit II, latency	3.2 ± .2 msec
Ulnar, wrist to digit V, latency	3.2 ± .25 msec
Sural (at 14 cm), lateral ankle-leg	3.5 ± .25 msec

COMPLICATIONS

The EMG and NCV studies are uncomfortable. However, the discomfort subsides immediately after the EMG needle is withdrawn or the electrostimulus has ended. As a rule, analgesics before, during or after the examination are not necessary. Tolerance to the two procedures varies among patients.

Clean technique is used in EMG needle insertion, except when the overlying skin is visibly dirty. An alcohol swab may be used to clean the skin. Sterile technique is not necessary. An EMG needle should be safely discarded if it is used in a patient suspected of Creutzfeldt-Jakob syndrome.

COMMON JARGON

Insertional activity is the oscilloscopic patterns related to the movement of the probing EMG needle in muscle. Increased insertional activity is nonspecific and is often observed in dysfunction of the primary motor unit.

Postinsertional activity follows the immediate cessation of needle movement in muscle. **Positive sharp waves** and bizarre high frequency discharges are pathologic and probably represent discharges from an irritable muscle fiber.

Two types of **spontaneous activity** may occur after insertional activity has subsided. **Fibrillations** have pathologic significance and represent abnormal muscle fiber activity as a result of an "irritation" of the primary motor unit. **Fasciculation** is the spontaneous twitching of a motor unit. This activity may be normal or abnormal, as in acute disease of the anterior horn cell.

Motor unit potential (MUP) is the action potential generated by motor unit activity and is measured in terms of its amplitude (microvolts), duration (milliseconds), and configuration (polyphasic is abnormal). Primary myopathic and neuropathic processes have their individual characteristic patterns of MUPs.

Recruitment represents the voluntary effort of the patient to mobilize motor units gradually and synchronously. The rate, quality, and quantity of MUPs generated by recruitment may reveal characteristic features of a primary myopathic or neuropathic process. Maximum recruitment may be limited by needle-induced pain as the muscle contracts or in patients who cannot respond to a command to contract.

Latency is the time (milliseconds) for the electrostimulus to travel from external stimulation to the muscle or sensory nerve. The response is detected by an active electrode overlying the muscle or sensory nerve. Sometimes the active electrode is a needle inserted into the muscle. For routine motor fiber evaluation, metal discs are usually preferred. For routine sensory fiber evaluation, elastic rings or metal discs are preferred.

Evoked response is the measured motor or sensory response to electrostimulation. Its amplitude is an important variable.

Repetitive stimulation is a technique utilized to evaluate the function of the neuromuscular junction. One method involves a train of 2–3 shocks per second over a 2- to 3-second period before and after a tetanic train or maximal voluntary isometric exercise of the muscle under evaluation. The different neuromuscular junction diseases have characteristic patterns.

INTERPRETATION

Axonal degeneration due to compression of the motor roots usually does not produce EMG abnormalities until the 3rd week (range, 14–28 days) in the upper or lower extremities. Thus, a "normal" or negative EMG study of a patient who clinically appears to have serious nerve impingment due to a herniated disc can be falsely negative if performed within 2 weeks of symptom onset.

A pathologic EMG pattern suggestive of muscle disease does not differentiate its etiology. Dystrophy, myositis, and myopathy share similar EMG abnormalities. As an exception, myotonic dystrophy has a characteristic sound and pattern.

Fibrillations and positive sharp waves reflect an irritation of muscle fiber. They never represent a normal condition and may be observed in most cases of acute dysfunction of the primary motor unit.

Motor or sensory fiber NCVs measure the health of myelinated peripheral nerves. However, severe axonal failure may secondarily influence myelin and thereby impair nerve conduction. Conversely, severe demyelinization can affect the axon.

A **negative** finding may not necessarily mean a **normal** finding. Limitations of the basic method, errors in measurement, background electrical interference, worn out needles, improper technique of electrode application, incomplete study, and an uncooperative patient may influence the results. False negatives are an inherent problem in electrodiagnosis but can be kept to a minimum.

Localized trauma from ordinary activity may produce pockets of positive sharp waves. If the sampled muscle has been subject to bumping, bruising, needle injections, or surgery, other muscles should be evaluated to corroborate the abnormal finding.

If a study is normal or negative, a follow-up study may prove to be invaluable in documenting physiologic changes in a suspected primary motor unit dysfunction.

REFERENCES

American Association of Electromyography and Electrodiagnosis, 732 Marquette Bank Building, Rochester, Minnesota 55901.

Goodgold J, Eberstein A: Electrodiagnosis of Neuromuscular Diseases, 3rd ed. Baltimore, Williams & Wilkins, 1983.

Johnson EW (ed): Practical Electromyography. Baltimore, Williams & Wilkins, 1980.

Smorto MP, Basmajian JV: Electrodiagnosis, A Handbook for Neurologists. Hagerstown, Harper & Row, 1977.

Sunderland SS: Nerves and Nerve Injuries, 2nd ed. New York, Churchill Livingstone, 1978.

32

CORTICOSTEROIDS FOR INJECTION INTO JOINT SPACE, BURSA, AND TENDON SHEATH

The single and cumulative dose of corticosteroid for any given patient varies with the degree of inflammation, the size of the anatomic pathology, and the relative response to overall therapy. Unlike their intravenous or oral forms, equivalent doses cannot be reliably approximated when the injection takes place in a bursa, tendon sheath, or joint space. As a rule, the relative anti-inflammatory potency of a corticosteroid preparation is based on cortisol (hydrocortisone), which has a potency value of 1.

Obviously, corticosteroid should **not** be injected into an area of **noninflammation** and should be repeated very judiciously because of the local catabolic effects on bone and soft tissue. Doses may be repeated every 5–7 days to 4–8 weeks as many as 3–4 times.

Many physicians prefer to mix the injected corticosteroid with lidocaine 1% or 2% (alternatively, procaine 1% or 2%) for its immediate local anesthetic effect against the burning of the corticosteroid solution. Other physicians think that its use is unnecessary for comfort.

Each physician has his or her preference of injectable corticosteroids. The list below represents frequently reported corticosteroids in the literature and by no means excludes other preparations.

Hydrocortisone acetate. Concentration of 25 mg/ml and 50 mg/ml. Relative potency = 1. Short half-life. Intra-articular absorption complete by 24–48 hours. Single dose for large joint, 25–50 mg; small joint, 10–25 mg; bursa, 25–50 mg; and tendon sheath, 5.0–12.5 mg.

Betamethasone sodium phosphate (Celestone) and **betamethasone** acetate (Soluspan) **mix.** In 1 ml, 3 mg of each drug is present. Relative potency = 25. Sodium phosphate form is rapid (1–3 hours) and acetate form is slow-acting (persists for 7 days). Effects may last for 1–2 weeks. Single dose for large joint is 6–12 mg (1–2 ml of mix); small joint, 1.5–6.0 mg (0.25–1.00 ml); bursa, 6 mg (1 ml); and tendon sheath, 1.5–3.0 mg (0.25–0.50 ml).

Methylprednisolone acetate (Depo-Medrol). Concentration at 20 mg/ml, 40 mg/ml, and 60 mg/ml. Relative potency = 5. Single dose for large joint is 20–80 mg; small joint, 4–40 mg; bursa 4–30 mg. Intra-articular absorption continues for 7 days.

Triamcinolone acetonide (Kenalog). Concentration at 10 mg/ml and 40 mg/ml. Relative potency = 5. Single dose for large joint is

15–40 mg; small joint, 2.5–10.0 mg; and tendon sheath, 2.5–10.0 mg.

Triamcinolone diacetate (Aristocort, Cenocort, and others). Concentration at 25 mg/ml and 40 mg/ml. Relative potency = 5. Single dose for large joint is 25 mg; small joint, 2–5 mg.

Triamcinolone hexacetonide (Aristospan). Concentration at 5 mg/ml and 20 mg/ml. Relative potency = 5. Single dose for large joint is 10–20 mg; small joint, 2–6 mg.

33

NONSTEROIDAL ANTI-INFLAMMATORY DRUGS

Every several years, new nonsteroidal anti-inflammatory drugs appear. The list below is a quick reference to older drugs for which there has been a greater experience in individual efficacy and adverse effects. There are, however, no clearly established relative anti-inflammatory potencies and comparable dose equivalencies as exist for oral or intravenous corticosteroids.

The following guidelines may be helpful in the prescription of nonsteroidal anti-inflammatory drugs:

1. Clinical indications for starting, continuing, or stopping should be understood by the physician.

2. Patient should be informed of frequent or major adverse effects.

3. Continued prescription is contingent on regular clinical or laboratory monitoring for progress, maintenance, or toxicity.

4. Dosage for rheumatoid arthritis may tend to be less than that for osteoarthritis or ankylosing spondylitis.

5. Drugs differ in their recommended initial doses. Some begin with higher doses and others with lower doses than the expected usual maintenance dosage.

6. The effect varies from 1–4 weeks but averages about 2 weeks after a maximal tolerable dose.

7. These drugs can be highly interactive with other medication and laboratory tests.

8. Many of the drugs are available only under their trade name.

DRUGS

Acetylsalicylic Acid. Average maintenance 2.4–3.6 g divided into q4- to 6-hour doses daily. Available in tabs (mg) at 75, 300, 325, 600, and 650; enteric-coated tabs (mg) at 300, 325, 350, 600, and 650; and buffered tabs (Ascriptin A/D, Bufferin) at 325 mg. Choline magnesium trisalicylate (Trilisate) comes in 500-mg tabs with average dose 3–4 g divided into Q4- to 6-hour doses daily.

Fenoprofen Calcium (Nalfon). Initial dose of 600 mg q.i.d. Usual maintenance of 1.2–2.4 g divided into 4 doses daily. Available in 300-mg capsule and 600-mg tablet.

Ibuprofen (Motrin). Usual maintenance of 1.2–2.4 g divided into 3–4 doses daily. Available in 300- and 400-mg tablets.

Indomethacin (Indocin). Initial dose of 25 mg b.i.d.–t.i.d. Usual maintenance of 100–200 mg divided into 2–4 doses daily. Response may vary between 1 and 4 weeks. Available in 25- and 50-mg capsules.

Naproxen (Naprosyn). Usual maintenance of 500–750 mg divided into 2 doses daily. Available in 250-mg tablet.

Phenylbutazone (Azolid, Butazolidin). Initial dose of 100–200 mg q8 hours. Usual maintenance of 100–400 mg divided into 3–4 doses daily. Available in 100-mg tablets.

Sulindac (Clinoril). Initial dose of 150–200 mg b.i.d. Usual maintenance of 300–400 mg divided into 2 doses daily. Available in 150- and 200-mg tablets.

Tolmetin Sodium (Tolectin). Initial dose of 400 mg t.i.d. Usual maintenance of 0.6–1.8 g divided into 3 doses daily. Available in 200-mg tablet with a sodium content of 18 mg.

REFERENCES

Hansten PD: Drug Interactions, 4th ed. Philadelphia, Lea & Febiger, 1979.

Physicians' Desk Reference, 37th ed. Oradell, N.J., Medical Economics, 1983.

Simon LS, Mills JA: Nonsteroidal antiinflammatory drugs, parts 1 and 2. New Engl J Med *302*:1179, 1237, 1980.

IV

SPECIFIC CHRONIC PHYSICAL DISABILITIES

34

SPINAL CORD INJURY

A **complete** injury involves the total loss of sensory **and** motor function below the level of injury. This usually can be determined at 72 hours after injury.

An **incomplete** injury means that there is partial preservation of sensory or motor, or both, functions below the level of injury. A common incomplete injury is the central cord syndrome, in which sensory function is better preserved and the lower extremities are stronger than the upper extremities.

With incomplete injury, the prognosis is extremely variable and impossible to predict early in the course. There may be only mild sensory sparing or nearly complete recovery. Approximately 50% of patients with incomplete cervical spinal cord injury will walk within 2 years of injury.

Level of injury is determined by careful neurologic examination and not by the level of bony dislocation or fracture. For example, a patient with a complete C5 quadriplegia has intact sensory **and** muscle function at spinal segment C5. The most common levels of injury are C5–6, T6–7, and T12–L1. Fifty percent of patients are quadriplegics; the other 50% are paraplegics.

ETIOLOGY AND INCIDENCE

In the United States, there are over 150,000 people with spinal cord injury. The incidence is 25–35 new cases per 100,000 people annually. Fifty percent are related to motor vehicle accidents; 15%, sports; 15%, falls; 10%, penetrating wounds; and 10%, other causes. Sixty percent of patients are from 15–29 years old at the time of injury; 30%, 30–59 years old; 5%, 60+ years old. Less than 5% of patients are under age 15 years at injury.

At the time of injury, 60% are employed; 10%, unemployed; 25%, students; and 5%, in other capacities. Sixty percent have their high school diploma or more. The other 40% have not graduated from high school. Fifty percent are single and 33% married at injury. Eighty percent of patients are males and only 20% are females.

ACUTE STAGE

Two to 12 weeks may lapse between the onset of spinal shock and the appearance of reflexes below the level of the injury.

Usually, autonomic and motor reflexes begin to appear within 6 weeks and may continue to change over the ensuing 2–6 months. Anal wink, bulbocavernosus, and Babinski reflexes are frequently the first to return.

Vertebral Column Instability. Most burst and compression fractures from direct loading are stable and need only external immobilization to decrease pain and allow healing. The greatest majority of fractures, however, are flexion-rotation injuries that require long immobilization in bed (8–12 weeks) or internal fixation and fusion. Adequate alignment is paramount to final long-term success, which usually means internal fixation and fusion.

If unstable, the cervical spine stability is achieved by bone grafting the area of instability. This is usually achieved best by wiring the posterior spinous processes and placing graft along the facets. It also may be achieved by anterior intervertebral block or strutt fusion. Thoracic and lumbar spine stability is achieved by Harrington rod fixation and bone grafting. Occasionally, Weiss springs are preferred over, or in addition to, Harrington rods.

External support is necessary after fusion. For the neck, the orthopedic surgeon or neurosurgeon may recommend a cervical collar or a rigid orthosis involving the head, neck, and trunk. These external supports limit the neck more effectively in the anterior-posterior direction than in lateral bend or rotation. At best, mobility may vary from 10–20% of normal sagittal movement, more than half of normal lateral bend, and a quarter of normal rotation. The SOMI (Sternal-Occipital-Mandibular-Immobilizer) and Four-poster Thomas Collar are widely recommended because of their overall comfort, safety, and relative effectiveness.

For thoracic and lumbar injuries, a form-fitted plastic body jacket is usually recommended. In the presence of a compression fracture of the vertebral body, a hyperextension orthosis is prescribed to specifically restrict flexion. These external supports are usually worn for 8–12 weeks after cervical fusion and 4–6 months after thoracic or lumbar spine fusion.

Spinal Shock. The total loss of all reflexes below the level of the injury continues 2–6 weeks before gradual return of autonomic and motor reflexes over 2–6 months. Anal wink, bulbocavernosus, and Babinski reflexes are usually the first to return.

Neurogenic Bladder. During spinal shock, the bladder will not empty and must be drained by an indwelling catheter or intermittent catheterization. This latter method is preferred because of the low incidence of infection, mucosal trauma, and stone formation.

Neurogenic Bowel. Serious fecal impaction may occur. An ileus, loss of rectal reflexes, poor food intake, and prolonged immobilization predispose the patient to constipation. A regular bowel program should be established early. Daily stool softeners and copious fluids are important. A rectal suppository followed by anorectal digital stimulation may be planned after breakfast or dinner to take advantage of the gastrocolic reflex.

Respiratory Insufficiency. Patients with high quadriplegia, C4 level and above, have severe restrictive lung impairment, partial loss of neck accessory muscles, and possible injury to the phrenic nerves. With less than 20–25% of the expected vital capacity, most patients will require assisted mechanical ventilation. Many patients with inadequate ventilation in the acute phase may develop sufficient strength to breathe independently within 1–3 months of injury. If the spinal segments C3, 4, 5 were destroyed, the phrenic nerves will be completely lost. The patient will need permanent 24-hour life support systems to survive.

Heterotopic Bone Formation. The formation of true bone in soft tissue occurs in 10–50% of spinal cord injured patients. The cause is unknown but is suspected to be secondary to the trauma of overstretching across joints. The more common sites are the hips, knees, elbows, and paralumbar regions. It usually occurs within 4 months of the injury. Its inflammatory presentation must be differentiated from deep venous thrombosis, fracture, deep infection, hemorrhage, and acute disorders of the joint.

A bone scan is a sensitive and reliable indicator of the presence, growth, and maturation of heterotopic bone formation. Earlier, serum alkaline phosphatase may be increased. Plain radiographs may be negative until the 2nd or 3rd week.

Heterotopic bone may ankylose a joint and predispose the patient to severe secondary muscle and joint contractures. Efforts to keep the affected joint mobilized should continue. **Etidronate disodium** has been recommended to reduce the incidence and growth of heterotopic ossification. The drug does **not** appear to dissolve mature lesions, delay healing of bony fractures, or predispose the patient to fractures from incidental trauma.

Etidronate disodium (Didronel) may be prescribed at 20 mg/kg body weight per day for 2 weeks, followed by 10 mg/kg per day for 10 weeks. The effect of treatment for more than 12 weeks or beyond 4 months of injury is not known. The drug is available in 200-mg tablets.

Asymptomatic hyperphosphatemia has been observed but does not by itself constitute a reason for discontinuation of the drug. Lower doses should be given in the presence of impaired renal function. Theoretically, high doses may produce hypocalcemia. Diarrhea or nausea may be lessened by two divided doses. The dose should be taken 2 hours after oral intake of high calcium-, magnesium-, iron-, or aluminum-containing food or medication.

Orthopedic consultation may be necessary once the heterotopic bone has matured and has created significant restriction in joint range. Partial resection may be recommended.

Postural Hypotension. Prolonged immobilization for 3 or more weeks and the loss of normal sympathetic control create a problem in postural hypotension in patients with spinal cord injury. If the patient has **not** been gradually brought to an upright position of sitting, later on, standing, he or she is likely to complain of lightheadedness, dizziness, and sudden weakness. The difference between systolic and diastolic blood pressure may be less than 20–25 mm Hg; the pulse may be tachycardiac; and the systolic reading may be relatively hypotensive.

The anticipation of postural hypotension should stimulate early preparation of the patient by maximizing the activity of the patient. Specific conditioning exercises may be prescribed, for example, for the upper extremities while the patient lies in bed. Leg wrapping or support hose and an abdominal binder may be worn to help maintain blood pressure as the patient begins to assume a sitting and standing posture. The patient may be secured to a **tilt table** 2–3 times a day. The angle of the tilt is gradually increased to 70–80° with a standing tolerance of 20–30 minutes. Occasionally, a patient with quadriplegia requires a low dose of ephedrine initially to minimize symptomatic drops in blood pressure.

Pressure Sores. Patients should be turned every 2 hours during strict bed rest or sleeping. In sitting, complete relief over the ischial tuberosities should occur faithfully every 15–30 minutes. Areas overlying the ischial tuberosities, sacrum, trochanters, heels, and occiput are at high risk for skin breakdown.

Venous Stasis. All patients with significant spinal cord injury will have venous stasis and mild fibrin clotting in the lower extremities. There is a 15–20% incidence of diagnosed thromboembolic disease of the deep veins. There is a 2–5% death rate from pulmonary emboli. Low-dose subcutaneous heparin, 5000–7000 units q12 hours, is recommended routinely by some physicians. Compression stockings for the lower extremities and elevated legs during supination should be generally ordered. Doppler ultrasound, radionuclide scanning, plethysmography, and other tests may be performed to evaluate a swollen limb for acute thrombophlebitis. Treatment should commence immediately with anticoagulation.

Contractures of Muscles and Joints. With prolonged bed rest, the patient is at great risk for contracturing of muscle and joint. The most common sites are the hip adductors, hip flexors, hamstrings, and gastrocnemius-soleus muscles in the lower extremities and the shoulder, elbow, wrist, and hand intrinsic muscles in the upper extremities. The appearance of spasticity will aggravate these deformities. Well-padded splints and manual joint range of motion should be implemented and closely supervised.

Hypercalciuria and Hypercalcemia. Hypercalciuria is invariably present in a patient with prolonged immobilization. The urinary calcium output is 2–7 times normal amounts. It is most impressive in the quadriplegic patient. Renal and bladder stones may develop. Adequate hydration with 1500 ml or more of urine output per 24 hours, absence of indwelling catheter, and antibiotic treatment for urinary tract infection can minimize the formation of stones.

Hypercalcemia is rare but should be suspected in a patient who is nauseated and vomiting. It can lead to a medical emergency if it is not diagnosed early. Treatment may be difficult but should consist of intravenous saline and furosemide to increase the output of calcium and to replace fluid volumes. Diuretics, oral salt tablets, and high fluid intake may be recommended by some physicians to maintain a high calcium urinary output. Etidronate disodium at 20 mg/kg of body weight per day may be effective in some patients in lowering bone turnover.

CHRONIC PHASE

Rehabilitative Prognosis

S2–4 Injury. The patients have varying degrees of problems with bowel and bladder function due to anal and urethral sphincter impairment. In general, they are completely independent in mobility and self-care.

L4–S1 Injury. The patients have a reflexive neurogenic bladder, insensate dermatomes, and paralyzed hip extensors and ankle plantar flexors. Hip abductors may be weak. A pair of ankle-foot orthoses may stabilize the ankles. Forearm crutches or canes are usually necessary for walking.

L2–3 Injury. The patients have a reflexive neurogenic bladder, a larger area of insensate dermatomes, and the additional paralysis of the quadriceps or knee extensors. Hip adductors may be weak. The patients may benefit greatly by the prescription of knee-ankle-foot orthoses to stabilize the knees and ankles and a pair of crutches, axillary or forearm, for independent ambulation. Self-care skills require some teaching before independent behavior is attained.

L1–2 Injury. The patients have the same problem with the bladder, bowel, and insensate skin. The hip flexors and other hip muscle groups are weak. Walking is very strenuous and often supplements wheelchair locomotion, the principal means of mobility for the patients. For those who can use knee-ankle-foot orthoses, a walker provides greater support and balance than crutches. Because of chronic sitting, the skin overlying the ischial tuberosities is at great risk for skin breakdown. The learning of self-care skills is more difficult for these patients, who are capable of independent living.

T7–12 Injury. The level of paraplegia has now involved the muscles of the back and abdomen. Trunk balance is compromised. Expiration is affected. Cough is weaker. The abdomen may protrude during inspiration. The patient is at greater risk for respiratory illness. It is a rare exception that the patient prefers knee-ankle-foot orthoses and a walker over a wheelchair for independent, safe, functional locomotion.

T1–6 Injury. These patients rely on the wheelchair as their principal means of locomotion but lack the trunk balance to perform "wheelies," negotiate curbs, or climb into their wheelchair easily should they fall out of it. Self-care is increasingly more difficult. Less mobility further increases the risk of serious skin breakdown over insensate, bony areas of the perineum and low midback.

C8–T1 Injury. These patients are quadriplegic. Hand function is weaker than normal. They can propel their own wheelchairs and perform independent transfers. Self-care, home-making, toileting, and driving can be independent. Despite the poor trunk balance and weak hands, many patients live productive lives without attendant care. Adaptive equipment, utensils, and wheelchairs can greatly facilitate function.

C6–7 Injury. These patients have elbow extension, supination, pronation, and wrist extension but only little finger strength and wrist flexion. They usually require some level of attendant care. A manual wheelchair can be propelled over a flat, firm, level, obstacle-free surface laboriously. A powered wheelchair can greatly enhance independent mobility. With the help of a rachet-type flexor hinge orthosis, these patients can write, type, manipulate small objects, dress upper extremities, and self-feed. A bed frame with hanging loops and an electric bed may facilitate partial lower extremity dressing. Transfers, bowel programs, bladder catheterization, condom application, and pressure releases usually require the assistance of an attendant. Driving a car or van can be accomplished with adaptive controls and special training.

C5–6 Injury. There is some abduction and rotation at the shoulders and weak elbow flexion. These patients can feed themselves with mobile arm supports (balanced forearm orthoses) and a splint for the wrist or hand. They can type and write slowly. A powered wheelchair provides independent locomotion. Attendant care is critical.

C4–5 Injury. There is no motor function except for head and neck motion. These patients must have their environments adapted to function with mouth or head control. With such control, these patients can drive a powered wheelchair and manipulate an environmental control system.

C1–4 Injury. There is profound paralysis at or below the neck. Paralysis of the hemidiaphragms necessitates external mechanical ventilation for life support. Attendant care is advisable 24 hours a day. Tongue-, lip-, cheek-, chin-, or head-controlled switches have interfaced these profoundly disabled patients to powered wheelchairs and environmental control systems. In certain patients with intact phrenic nerves, radio frequency phrenic nerve pacers may be implanted and produce partial to complete removal of external mechanical ventilators.

Vertebral Instability. Even after a successful fusion of the back, Harrington rods may break or loosen and require removal. With the incomplete fusion and an angulation greater than 30 degrees, a secondary procedure is usually recommended to prevent progression.

Pneumonia. Beyond the acute phase, patients with quadriplegia or paraplegia above T10–12 are at risk for recurrent atelectasis and pneumonia. There are specific ways of reducing this risk. The patient with quadriplegia may be taught glossopharyngeal breathing by a speech pathologist. A responsible, well-trained attendant may perform "quad coughs" without risk of a rib fracture and secondary splenic rupture. Incentive inspirometers may be used. An abdominal corset may be worn to maintain intra-abdominal pressure during sitting. Without the corset, the flaccid abdominal wall pouches out and makes diaphragmatic breathing less effective in sitting. A pneumobelt consists of a broad rubber diaphragm that is placed across the abdomen. It is connected to a compressor that inflates it to assist expiration and deflates it to aid passive inspiration. Influenza vaccination should be given annually in early fall to high-risk patients.

Diagnostically, a chest film may be necessary to augment physical examination. Unless the patient has a chronic tracheostomy, sputum for Gram stain and culture is difficult to obtain from the ailing patient. Antibiotics should be prescribed, particularly when a history of aspiration is elicited.

Anesthetic Risk. There are many potentially **preventable** complications associated with general anesthesia in patients with acute or chronic spinal cord injury. The physician should discuss these potential complications with the anesthesiologist and surgeon:

A. **Pressure sore.** Prolonged lying on a hard or inadequately padded table in the operating room may lead to significant breakdown of skin. The occiput, scapulae, elbows, dorsal spinal processes, sacrum, pelvis, trochanters, knees, heels, and malleoli are at high risk for breakdown. The patient should be well padded and, if necessary, be lifted every 30–45 minutes for pressure relief. The skin should be carefully inspected before and after surgery.

B. **Autonomic dysreflexia.**

C. **Atelectasis, pneumonia, or ventilatory failure** may occur that is due to restrictive lung function, weak respiratory musculature, and aspiration. In general, elective surgery should be postponed in a patient with even mild respiratory symptoms.

D. **Hypotension and bradycardia** are thought to be due to the dysfunction in the autonomic nervous system. Analgesics, sedatives, and anesthetics may aggravate these symptoms and thus should be administered in relatively low doses.

E. **Succinylcholine toxicity.** In the presence of denervated muscle, succinylcholine can provoke a massive depolarization of muscle membrane and release of intracellular potassium. The resultant hyperkalemia can be fatal. **Cardiac irritability** may occur within minutes after intravenous succinylcholine infusion and lead to **cardiac arrest.** To be cautious, this drug is contraindicated between the 6th day and 6th month following spinal cord injury. However, in **this condition and others with acute or chronic denervation,** only **nondepolarizing anesthetic agents** should be employed.*

Chronic Pain. There are three sources of chronic pain or discomfort that often are not relieved by medication and may lead to classic operant behavior.

A. **Dysesthesias** are described as burning, tingling, aching, or numbing discomfort. It is postulated that dysesthesias arise from injured neural tissue or from a lack of thalamic inhibition of normal afferent sensation. Symptoms are perceived below the level of spinal cord injury.

B. **Dermatomal pain** is thought to be due to injury to nerve roots. Patients complain of sharp, shooting, stabbing pain or burning that follows a dermatomal pattern in its radiation. Although symptoms appear within a month of injury and usually subside within 3–6 months, they may persist, particularly in patients with injury to the cauda equina or low spinal cord.

C. **Visceral pain** may be described as vague, diffuse, deep pressure; cramping; or discomfort in the "back," "belly," "side," or "chest." Flatulence, nausea, and symptoms of autonomic dysreflexia may accompany it. Its appearance may or may not be clearly related to acute problems with the stomach, bladder, rectum, colon, or other viscus organs. Its pathophysiology is unknown.

The incidence of pain ranges from a third to all patients with spinal cord injury. Roughly three quarters of patients note the onset within 12 months of injury. The rate is higher in patients with lumbosacral injuries than in those with high thoracic or cervical lesions.

The management of chronic pain is eclectic: relaxation, self-hypnosis, psychotherapy, biofeedback, and transcutaneous electrical nerve stimulation. Over **sensate** skin, heat therapy has been applied with variable outcome. Analgesics, sedatives, tranquilizers, antiseizure drugs, and muscle relaxants have been prescribed. If a drug is tried, specific clinical indications for its use and continuation should be agreed to by the patient. The drug should be given on a time-contingent basis and not taken "only as necessary." Narcotics and other abusive substances should be avoided, if possible. A fifth to a third of symptomatic patients may complain of the severe, disabling effect chronic pain has on their life. Operant pain behavior is a real complication and can be minimized in these more severely affected patients by using sound psychologic principles.

Impaired thermoregulation may be seen in patients with spinal cord lesions above T8 and particularly at the cervical level. Patients become poikilothermic. Adjustment to cooler or warmer ambient temperatures is low, inconsistent, or aided by the amount of cover over the patient. For the severely disabled patients, periodic

---

*Brooke MM, Donovan WH, Stolov WC: Paraplegia: succinylcholine-induced hyperkalemia and cardiac arrest. Arch Phys Med Rehabil 59:306, 1978.

monitoring of the core temperature should occur during the day and especially when there is suspected inflammatory illness. Because of the severance of autonomic system pathways to the hypothalamus, cooling is not met with vasoconstriction and shivering and warming is not countered by vasodilation and perspiration.

Hypothermia or hyperthermia due to changes in ambient temperature responds within 1–3 hours of attendant care. Elevated temperature from infection, however, usually persists or recurs frequently despite efforts to cool the patient. Antipyretics have variable influence on fevers and work best in the less disabled patients.

Diaphoresis. The spinal sympathetic nervous system may be isolated from the influence of supraspinal centers in a patient with complete spinal cord injury. Excessive sweating may be particularly a problem in patients with low cervical cord injuries and is usually not observed in injuries below T8–10. Normal sweating occurs above the level of spinal cord injury. This diaphoresis occurs reflexively and is not part of the body's central thermoregulation for cooling.

Diaphoresis may be triggered by many different stimuli, such as bladder irritability, rectal distention, skin breakdown, urine infection, cellulitis, or alteration in bodily position. Diaphoresis may be associated with autonomic dysreflexia.

The sweating may present with an annoying hygienic problem and require frequent changing or cleaning of clothes, bed linen, and wheelchair cushions. The moist skin may be predisposed to fungal or bacterial superinfection, intertriginous rash, and breakdown from pressure, shear, or tissue distortion. Propantheline (Pro-Banthine) may be tried but is seldom effective over a long period. Minimizing aggravating factors constitutes optimal management.

Acute Surgical or Medical Abdomen. Cholelithiasis, pancreatitis, appendicitis, peritonitis, perforated ulcer, bowel obstruction, ruptured spleen, ureteral obstruction, and other acute conditions may be difficult to diagnose. A **high index of suspicion** is important in the examination of a patient with high paraplegia or quadriplegia.

Symptoms are often vague and consist of anorexia, nausea, vomiting, flatulence, malaise, fever, and chills. On examination, the patient may have signs of tachycardia, bradycardia, hypertension, hypotension, tachypnea, elevated temperature, increased spasm, abdominal rigidity, or shock. Localization of discomfort is frequently deep and diffuse to the abdomen with back or chest discomfort suggestive of referred pain. Laboratory and radiologic procedures are often nonspecific.

Prompt surgical consultation and frequent follow-up may be necessary to evaluate the patient for an acute surgical abdomen. Final diagnosis and treatment, however, may require an emergency laparotomy.

Fracture of osteoporotic long bones occurs at a high rate in patients with paraplegia or quadriplegia of long standing. The femur and tibia are most commonly fractured by often incidental or minor trauma during routine transfers, falling from a wheelchair, bumping against furniture, and other otherwise "insignificant" events. The application of a plaster circular cast should be followed closely because of the great and, at times absolute, risk of skin breakdown over insensate skin. A semirigid or soft splint and a well-padded bivalved cast are two alternative methods for bone healing. Frequent changes or inspections are desirable.

Management of the neurogenic bladder, neurogenic bowel, pressure ulcers, spasticity, autonomic dysreflexia, contractures, sexual dysfunction, and psychologic adjustment is discussed in detail elsewhere in this manual.

REFERENCES

Donovan WH, Bedbrook SG: Comprehensive Management of Spinal Cord Injury. CIBA Clinical Symposia. *34*(2), 1982.

Ford JR, Duckworth B: Physical Management for the Quadriplegic Patient. Philadelphia, FA Davis, 1974.

Handbook for Paraplegic and Quadriplegic Individuals. The National Spinal Cord Injury Foundation, 369 Elliot Street, Newton Upper Falls, Massachusetts 02164.

Kewalramani LS: Ectopic ossification. Am J Phys Med 56:99, 1977.

Pierce DS, Nickel VH: The Total Care of Spinal Cord Injuries. Boston, Little Brown, 1977.

Yashon D: Spinal Injury. New York, Appleton-Century-Crofts, 1978.

Young JS, Burns PE, Bowen AM, McCutchen R: Spinal Cord Injury Statistics. Phoenix, Good Samaritan Medical Center, 1982.

35

CEREBROVASCULAR ACCIDENTS

Cerebrovascular accidents (CVAs) are the result of obstruction or rupture of cerebral or brainstem arteries, producing loss in central nervous system function. Motor control, sensation, and cognition may be profoundly affected.

There are three general categories of CVAs. Thrombosis accounts for two thirds to three quarters of cerebrovascular accidents. A fifth to a quarter are due to intracerebral or subarachnoid hemorrhage. Five to 15% result from emboli most commonly related to cardiac or carotid vasculature disorders.

Functional impairment varies widely and may involve walking, self-care, communication, vision, judgment, memory, cognition, behavior, emotional stability, and psychosocial adjustment.

PROGNOSIS

In the United States, over 2 million people are disabled by CVAs. Its incidence is highest between 50 and 80 years of age, with a rate 2–3 times greater in the group above 65 years. Under age 60, its occurrence is slightly greater in males than in females.

Prognosis for surviving and returning home is associated with the following characteristics: no predisposing factors such as hypertension, hyperlipidemia, cardiac valvular disease, diabetes, previous stroke; under age 60–65 years; minimal or no loss of consciousness at onset; mild or absent aphasia; medically stable and improving at 4 weeks; and supportive family. Because of unilateral neglect and visual-spatial perceptual deficits, the prognosis for patients with left hemiplegia may be less optimistic than for patients with right hemiplegia. Under age 50, the prospects of return to work are brighter than for the group over age 50.

IMPAIRED MOBILITY

If voluntary activity appears within the 1st week, nearly 9 of every 10 patients can eventually walk safely, independently, and functionally. If voluntary motor recovery commences between the 1st and 4th weeks, eventual independent ambulation develops in two thirds to three quarters of patients. Particularly for moderate to long distances, the wheelchair becomes the principal means of locomotion. A patient is appropriate for limited ambulation training if he or she has satisfactory standing balance; is free from deforming contractures at the hip, knee, or ankle; can selectively control movement at those joints; and can follow directions through verbal or nonverbal communication.

Progression of an ambulation program should be gradual, be success-oriented, and await mastery of each motoric step. The patient should shift weight over the involved extremity well before advancing to a single or double bar setup. An even, symmetric, stable walk should be learned before the use of a quad cane. Finally, the replacement of the quad cane with a single point cane should await a consistently stable gait.

A plastic or metal ankle-foot orthosis is frequently prescribed for the patient to stabilize the involved ankle, discourage genu recurvatum, and make walking more energy efficient.

Functional electrical stimulation may be appropriate for hemiplegic patients with the following characteristics: minimal or no contractures at the hip, knee, or ankle; absent overpowering equinovalgus; mild to moderate weakness in the muscle groups; peroneal nerve responsive to usual levels of stimulating current; and, most important, an appropriate comprehension of the system. Functional electrical stimulation is utilized as a therapeutic tool during training sessions.

SELF-CARE

The patient may initially require help in dressing, undressing, grooming, hygiene, and toileting. An occupational therapist may teach the patient special techniques in overcoming poor motor control in a limb. Special utensils may aid self-feeding; adaptive clothing may facilitate dressing or undressing; grab bars may make toileting safer; a shower extension and tub bench may make bathing efficient. For the patient who progresses, kitchen activities may be important to evaluate and teach.

NEGLECT

Particularly in a patient with a classic right hemispheric CVA, the phenomenon of neglect may be observed. The patient with left hemiplegia tends to ignore the left side despite sensory stimuli, such as vision, hearing, or touch. For example, the patient may ignore the meal, cards, or magazine on the left side of the table and attend entirely to the right side. The left arm and leg are "forgotten" in self-care and mobility. Neglect may be aggravated by the presence of a visual field cut.

VISUAL PERCEPTUAL IMPAIRMENT

Dysfunction of the right hemisphere, which is thought to process nonlanguage stimuli, may result in a lack of spatial perception and in understanding that a "piece" may be part of a meaningful "whole." In self-care, for example, a sleeve, buckle, button, or pocket may not be processed as part of a shirt, belt, or pants. In reading, a paragraph, column, chapter, or photograph may not be comprehended as part of a page, table, book, or description.

DYSPHAGIA

In bilateral or brainstem CVAs, dysphagia is commonly observed and can precipitate aspiration. If the situation is acute, tracheal intubation and a feeding tube may be required. If the patient is alert, has a gag reflex, coughs well, and handles ice chips without choking, Jello, custard, and other foodstuffs that do not separate easily may be introduced. The patient should never eat with the head in hyperextension. A speech pathologist may be consulted to assess a patient's dysphagia. Most rehabilitative occupational therapists can perform a limited evaluation and recommend a safe progression of food items.

A barium swallow and otolaryngologic consultation may be necessary to evaluate the musculature (facial, pharyngeal, lingual, laryngeal, esophageal) of chewing and swallowing. In unusual cases, a surgeon may need to perform a feeding gastrostomy, esophagostomy, or jejunostomy for prolonged severe dysphagia.

COMMUNICATION

Dysarthria, aphasia, apraxia, and other abnormalities of communication may result from CVAs. In patients with left hemiplegia, communication should be simple, concrete, direct, and repetitious. In patients with right hemiplegia, however, the emphasis of communication should be through gesticulation, pantomime, and other clearly demonstrable physical activity before the patient. In practice, people should communicate in a quiet environment and try both methods simultaneously. The consultation of a speech pathologist and psychologist is important.

PSYCHOLOGIC COMPLICATIONS

Careful observations and standardized testing best describe a patient's psychologic problems. Memory, spatial perception, perseveration, and depression may be observed. A clinical psychologist or neuropsychologist should be consulted.

Lists, cards, posters, schedules, calendars, and pictures are excellent forms of cues that help the patient recall and attend to a structured program.

For spatial-perceptual deficits, the environment should be modified to minimize distraction. Improvement may be slow and impede a patient's independence.

Perseveration is a tendency to utilize an involuntary verbal and motor response that persists inappropriately. Simple verbal commands or changing the subject may effectively help the patient deal with perseveration.

The behavioral appearance of depression occurs in many patients recovering from a CVA. To what extent the depressive symptoms reflect a neurophysiologic dysfunction is not clear. It is thought that depression in the patient with left hemiplegia is due to failure and frustration to attain basically unrealistic goals. In the patient with a right hemiplegia, however, depression is said to be a hyperreaction to a self-awareness that there are "insurmountable" disabilities to overcome. Antidepressants may be prescribed in selective cases.

Graphs, videotape replays, and generous praise are ways to provide direct, supportive feedback to the discouraged, depressed patient. Psychiatric consultation, however, may be necessary, particularly if the patient has a positive family or premorbid history of primary depression.

SEIZURES

Although seizures occur more frequently with hemorrhagic than ischemic lesions, **late onset seizures** may occur, usually within the 1st year, in a wide variety of stroke syndromes. An episode may be precipitated by fatigue, intercurrent illness, and other stresses.

SHOULDER PAIN

Subluxation of the glenohumeral joint occurs when there is shoulder laxity due to flaccid hemiplegia. Capsular and rotator cuff tears occur frequently and may be precipitated by excessive range of motion at the shoulder joint. Inadvertent or careless banging of the flaccid shoulder and arm is more likely to happen in patients who neglect the affected side. Brachial plexus injuries may result from similar causes and may be suspected when the wrist, hand, or fingers tend to recover faster than the proximal shoulder and elbow. Shoulder-hand syndrome can also occur.

Electrodiagnosis is a useful tool in screening a hemiplegic upper extremity for a brachial plexus injury. Although management will continue to be palliative or supportive, the expectation of recovery may be significantly modified.

If an extremity is flail, it should be protected from injury and glenohumeral subluxation. Under optimal conditions, the support should counter the pull of gravity and hold the humerus in the shoulder joint. Views differ on the use of slings. Some recommend that the arm be stabilized by having the patient keep the hand in his or her pants pocket while standing or walking. Sitting in a wheelchair, the patient may place the affected arm on the lap tray with the hand positioned toward the middle or center. Others prefer that the arm be placed in an armrest trough. Lying in bed, the patient may support the involved extremity with a pillow.

The shoulder should receive daily range of motion exercises to minimize contractures of muscles and joints. Many patients can be taught to perform range of motion using the contralateral, unaffected arm for active assistance. Ultrasound and vigorous static stretch may be necessary. **Adhesive capsulitis** (so-called frozen shoulder) is a dreaded complication seen in acquired hemiplegia. Its incidence, however, can be significantly lowered with an early, vigorous program of therapy.

URINARY INCONTINENCE

Urinary incontinence in the acute phase of a CVA is usually due to a lack of inhibition. Urination may be frequent, small in volume, and precipitate. In a typical situation, a cystometrogram is generally unnecessary. As the patient recovers, greater inhibition develops and the sense of urgency begins to diminish. Fluid intake may be balanced over the day and restricted after dinner. The patient may be asked to void as frequently as every 2–3 hours. In some situations, an anticholinergic may be effective but is generally not necessary. For the night time or in difficult male patients, a condom catheter may be recommended. Indwelling catheters should be avoided. Accessibility to a urinal, bedpan, bedside commode, or toilet is important and is often a problem at home. A home visit may be recommended to assess safety, transfers, and accessibility to the bathroom.

STOOL INCONTINENCE

Fecal soiling is a poor prognostic sign in the rehabilitation of a patient. A bowel program should be established early in the patient's course and prescribed for home, if necessary.

SOCIAL AND VOCATIONAL ISSUES

A social worker or vocational counselor may be requested to assess the patient's potential to work again or live at home. There are consumer support organizations, visiting nurse associations, home meal deliveries, and housing for disabled elderly people.

The patient's work capability depends largely on the nature of the CVA, the clinical progress, and the patient's premorbid attributes.

CLASSIC RIGHT AND LEFT HEMISPHERIC SYNDROMES

Right Cerebrovascular Accident. The patient has left hemiplegia and impairment in the following: visual and spatial perception; processing of nonlanguage data; comprehending the "whole" from one or more of its "parts"; left-sided neglect; left hemianopsia; and awareness of his or her newly acquired deficits. Verbal communication may be preferred.

Left Cerebrovascular Accident. The patient has right hemiplegia and problems with the following: aphasia; high anxiety; disorganization; depression from excessive "sensitivity" to the multiple deficits; and right hemianopsia. Pantomime may be more effective than spoken language.

REFERENCES

Anderson TP, Bourestom NM, Greenberg PR, Hildyard V: Predictive factors in stroke rehabilitation. Arch Phys Med Rehabil 55:545, 1974.

Chaco W: Subluxation of the glenohumeral joint in hemiplegia. Am J Phys Med 50:139, 1971.

Fowler RS, Fordyce WE: Stroke patients, why do they behave that way? Dallas, American Heart Association, 1974.

Griffin J, Reddin G: Shoulder pain in patients with hemiplegia. Phys Ther 61:1041, 1981.

Lehmann JF, et al: Stroke rehabilitation, outcome and prediction. Arch Phys Med Rehabil 56:383, 1975.

Moskowitz E: Complications in the rehabilitation of hemiplegic patients. Med Clin North Am 53:541, 1969.

Moskowitz E, Porter JI: Peripheral nerve lesions in upper extremity in hemiplegic patients. New Engl J Med 269:776, 1973.

Mossman PL: A Problem Oriented Approach to Stroke Rehabilitation. Springfield, Ill., Charles C Thomas, 1976.

Renshaw DC: Stroke and Sex, pp 121–132. In Comfort A: Sexual Consequences of Disability. Philadelphia, George Stickley, 1978.

Sier E, Freishtat B: Perceptual Dysfunction in the Adult Stroke Patient, a Manual for Evaluation and Treatment. Boston, Charles B Slack, 1976.

Weisbroth S, Esibill N, Zuger RR: Factors in the vocational success of hemiplegic patients. Arch Phys Med Rehabil 52:441, 1971.

36

CLOSED HEAD INJURY

Closed head injury is the most common civilian head injury. The mechanism of injury usually involves a blunt object that strikes the head or a head that hits a hard surface. Momentum is imparted to the head, with a resultant diffuse shearing of white matter fiber. Thus, deficits can often be scattered and selective.

A **concussion** is an immediate loss of consciousness. Neuronal dysfunction is transient and reversible with resolution within minutes to hours of injury. In most cases, loss of consciousness and post-traumatic amnesia usually resolve within 12 hours. Attention, however, has been given to protracted irritability, insomnia, lack of concentration, and depression after concussions in otherwise neurologically healthy people who have suffered concussion.

A **contusion** involves an immediate loss of consciousness due to neuronal injury, which is partly reversible over days to months. Loss of consciousness and post-traumatic amnesia usually last more than 24 hours.

The closed head injury may be associated with depressed skull fracture; intracerebral, subdural, or epidural hemorrhage; or tentorial herniation.

Unlike closed head injury, penetrating head injury occurs from missiles, such as bullets or fragments from exploding objects. Consciousness may be preserved if a tiny object penetrates the brain at a relatively low velocity. Focal neurologic symptoms and post-traumatic epilepsy are more common in penetrating injuries.

The annual incidence of all head injuries is 40 per 1000 people in the United States. Severe head injuries occur at a rate of 2–10 per 1000 people. Males outnumber females 3 to 1. The risk is greater among children 4–5, males 15–24, the elderly, and people who have had head injuries previously. The mortality, however, is higher in adults than in children. Motor vehicle accidents, falls, job-related accidents, recreational accidents (e.g., golf, horseback riding, football), and assault constitute the more frequent causes of head injury.

INITIAL EVALUATION AND PROGNOSIS

Depth of Coma

The **depth** of coma may be assessed by the Glasglow Coma Scale (Table 36–1).

Table 36–1. GLASGLOW COMA SCALE

EYES	Open	Spontaneously	4
		To speech or verbal command	3
		To pain	2
	No response		1
BEST MOTOR RESPONSE	To verbal command	Obeys	6
	To painful stimulus	Localizes pain	5
		Withdrawal	4
		Abnormal flexion (decorticate rigidity)	3
		Extension (decerebrate rigidity)	2
		No response	1
BEST VERBAL RESPONSE		Oriented	5
		Confused conversation	4
		Inappropriate words	3
		Incomprehensible sounds	2
		No response	1
Total			Range of 3–15

The sum of the cumulative responses may be as low as 3 and as high as 15. The examiner's knuckles may be applied to the patient's sternum for a nociceptive stimulus. To assess verbal response, the examiner may need to arouse the patient with a painful stimulus.*

Forty to 50% of patients will be dead or vegetative at 6 months postinjury if they fail to open their eyes, obey verbal commands, or speak words within 6 hours. Death or a vegetative state is highly probable if the patient shows abnormal motor response (decerebrate or absent motor response to pain), impaired ocular cephalic or vestibular reflexes, and impaired pupillary responses bilaterally for 72 hours or more.

Duration of Coma

Survival. When adults and children are decerebrate for 3 months or more, death or a vegetative state is likely.

Ambulation. In adolescents and young adults, decerebration for less than 24 hours and post-traumatic amnesia for less than 2 months are associated with independent ambulation. For middle-aged and elderly patients, an absence of decerebration and post-traumatic amnesia under 2 weeks are predictive of walking independently. However, coma of 8–13 weeks or more is associated with dependent mobility.

---

*Teasdale G, Jennett B: Assessment of coma and impaired consciousness: practical scale. Lancet 2:81, 1974.

Self-Care. One study showed that when coma persisted beyond 24 hours, 73% of children and adolescents were independent in self-care at 1 year; 10%, partly independent; and 17%, totally dependent. When coma lasted beyond 48 hours, 51% of adults with closed head injury were independent in self-care; 37%, partly independent; and 12%, totally dependent. The likelihood of full self-care was lower when coma exceeded 12 weeks, systolic hypertension appeared between days 1 and 3 postinjury, and the cerebral ventricles were enlarged on CT scan, usually within 2 weeks.

Mental Function. Despite complete physical recovery, more than 30% of children with coma less than an hour manifested subsequent behavioral problems. When coma persisted beyond 24 hours, nearly 50% of patients with independent walking and self-care demonstrated severe emotional disturbances, such as impulsivity, low frustration tolerance, emotional lability, social withdrawal, and phobias. Psychologic counseling was necessary.

Employability. When coma lasted between 1 and 7 days, 80% of adults with closed head injury later became employed. When coma lasted between 1 and 4 weeks, less than 50% held jobs at follow-up. When coma persisted beyond 4 weeks, less than 20% were eventually employed.

Post-Traumatic Amnesia

The duration of post-traumatic amnesia is the period during which continuous memory is absent. This period may be roughly estimated by asking the patient about his or her first and subsequent memories after the injury. The post-traumatic amnesia ends when the patient exhibits recall of continuous events from day to day. Another method is based on the patient's daily performance on a recall task. When the patient accomplishes the task on 2 or more consecutive days, the post-traumatic amnesia has ended.

The duration of post-traumatic amnesia appears to be a stronger predictor of eventual learning capacity than is the duration of coma. A moderate amount of cognitive dysfunction is associated with a post-traumatic amnesia 2–8 weeks in duration in adolescents and young adults. In middle-aged and elderly patients, severe cognitive impairment is associated with post-traumatic amnesia of 4 weeks or more.

When this period is less than an hour, 95% of patients will resume employment in 2 months. When the period exceeds 24 hours, the rate falls to 80% within 6 months postinjury. When coma or post-traumatic amnesia is 1 week or longer, 37% of patients die soon or remain in a vegetative state.

Speech and Language

In a studied population of patients with closed head injury in an inpatient rehabilitation setting, 32% of patients manifested aphasia and 38% dysarthria. Deficits in naming, fluency, and reading were noted in the other 30% of patients. In another population, 24% of patients exhibited aphasia at 4 months and 16% at 3 years.

Employability

Employability correlates best with the level of mental function. Sixty-two percent of patients with no or mild mental changes were employed by follow-up. Among patients with moderate to severe mental changes, only 23% held jobs. The probability of employment was diminished by deficits in speech or language, severe lack of motor control, age of 45 years or more, history of alcohol or drug abuse, and unstable premorbid personality.

Prognostic statements made before 3 months postinjury are less accurate. The most dramatic recovery occurs during the first 6 months. It is common opinion that neurologic recovery continues for several years. From the standpoint of rehabilitation, however, the patient's new learning capacity and adaptive skills are important prognostic markers at 1 year postinjury. In summary, the patient's age, the coma (depth and duration), and the post-traumatic amnesia (duration) are major predictors of functional outcome for patients with closed head injury.

MANAGEMENT OF INPATIENT REHABILITATION

Medical

Five percent of all hospitalized patients develop **late onset seizures,** which occur within the 1st year of injury in over half the cases. Sixty percent are generalized; 40%, focal.

The risk of late seizures (7 + days postinjury) is increased when coma is more than 24 hours; post-traumatic amnesia lasts more than 24 hours; dura is penetrated by trauma or surgery (e.g., depressed skull fracture, hematoma); focal neurologic signs are present; and seizures appear within the 1st week of injury. The risk may be as high as 60% when three or more of these factors are present. In general, individual risks of late seizures run 15–25%.

The prescription of antiseizure medication, such as phenytoin, is controversial. When two or more of these risk factors are present, many physicians recommend 2 years of prophylaxis. Hypoglycemia, fatigue, or alcoholism can precipitate seizures. If the patient has remained seizure-free for those 2 years, medication may be tapered off. Electroencephalograms can be insensitive indicators of whether the medication should be stopped or continued. The patient should be aware that the drug may have to be reinstituted if seizures recur.

Phenytoin 300–400 mg P.O. once daily or divided into two doses is the drug of choice. Its sedative effect is usually transient. Periodic blood levels should be taken to avoid inadvertent phenytoin intoxication (levels over 20 mcg/ml) or excessively low levels of less than 5–10 mcg/ml. As is true with other medications, a deterioration in performance may be due to phenytoin overdose. Symptoms may be characterized by ataxia, nystagmus, dysarthria, tremor, nausea, confusion, and somnolence.

Carbamazepine 200 mg P.O. t.i.d.–q.i.d. is an alternative should the patient show an intolerance or allergy to phenytoin. Starting dose is 200 mg daily or b.i.d. until a therapeutic maintenance dose is reached. It ranges between 800 and 1000 mg daily.

Post-traumatic **hydrocephalus** is suggested by a gradual deterioration in cognitive or motor function in a patient who had shown steady recovery or previously had been stable. Serial CT scans may reveal progressive ventricular enlargement in addition to or from other than cortical atrophy. A neurosurgeon should be consulted and the patient considered a candidate for a ventriculoperitoneal shunt. Normal pressure hydrocephalus, however, appears to respond less favorably to shunting.

Shoulder subluxation may result from weak shoulder abduction, which allows gravity and the momentum of limb movement to stretch the glenohumeral joint capsule. Pain and limited range of motion may result. An arm sling, wheelchair trough, or lap tray may minimize the problem.

Post-traumatic **action tremor** may appear with fine, careful, or rapid movements. This is different from the resting tremor of parkinsonian syndrome or the end point tremor of cerebellar dysfunction. Propranolol may be prescribed for the action tremor.

Heterotopic bone formation may occur in patients within the first 2 months of trauma, especially over the shoulders and hips. The use of etidronate disodium is not well established as a routine prophylaxis in this patient population.

Miscellaneous: Anosmia, diplopia, and visual field defects may be observed. Diabetes insipidus and hypothalamic hyperphagia have been known to last up to several months and are usually transient. Abuse of alcohol or drugs, deviant sexual behavior, and criminal acts have occurred following head injury. Suicidal behavior occurs and may appear within 6–12 months after the patient has been discharged from a supportive, structured inpatient rehabilitative program.

Criteria for Inpatient Rehabilitation

A. Score of 9 (Glasglow Coma Scale) within 3 months of injury.

B. Reliable rudimentary communication skills, such as 80% accuracy in responding to yes-no questions or following 8 out of 10 verbal, concrete, single-stage commands to perform.

C. Physical disability may be minimal or absent but the patient exhibits cognitive deficits that are likely to impede his or her recovery at home and in the community.

D. Highly structured, supportive behavioral mangement is desirable in decreasing patient's socially inappropriate behavior and in substituting prosocial behavior.

E. Neurologic and musculoskeletal recovery suggests important functional gains with proper teaching, adaptive equipment, walking aids, and other interventions.

F. The level and management of communication require evaluation, intervention, and re-evaluation.

G. Family needs teaching and training. Community-based services require planning and involvement prior to hospital discharge.

H. The complexity of the patient's case lends itself to a comprehensive, multidisciplinary team, which can expedite, facilitate, or more efficiently implement discharge.

PSYCHOLOGIC MANAGEMENT

A neuropsychologist and a behavioral psychologist complement each other well in the psychologic management of a patient with brain injury. Both consultants often recommend detailed flow charts of specific behaviors to describe the patient's behavior. There is often some overlap between the two fields in the use of standardized tests to measure mental function.

For a complete neuropsychologic assessment, the **Halstead-Reitan Neuropsychological Test Battery** may be recommended. It requires multiple testing sessions and often takes several hours to complete in a "cooperative" patient. Unlike conventional neurologic tests, this battery assesses language, perception, memory, attention, comprehension, abstraction, orientation (time and space), emotional status, verbal function, fluency, arithmetic, reading, sequencing, fine motor coordination, and other areas.

Components of the battery may be selectively repeated to follow the patient's progress. Deficits in one or more of these areas may explain the patient's recovery course and suggest specific strategies for cognitive retraining.

In setting goals, the physician may consider the following objectives in psychologic management: In **cognition,** the patient should learn to predict consequences; organize simple information; shift flexibly between 2 or 3 aspects of a situation; and intregrate information from one sensory modality with that of a second sensory modality efficiently.

In **behavior,** the patient learns to utilize appropriate social routines in appropriate situations and to inhibit inappropriate social, aggressive, or depressive responses.

In **language,** the patient should learn to use words intentionally and avoid perseveration. A reduction in aphasia or dysphasia is always highly desirable.

Affectively, the patient should learn to reduce wide swings in emotions, to control outbursts, and to curb periods of excessive agitation.

The professional staff should enlist the help of the family to provide the structure, support, orientation, consistency, calmness, and milieu in which the patient may relearn important social skills.

Perceptual deficits require evaluation and monitoring. Senses unaffected by agnosia should be utilized. If verbal memory or comprehension is impaired, gestures or pantomime are recommended. If verbal skills are intact, simple written instructions are desirable.

Memory should be followed with serial examinations. Deterioration may represent post-traumatic hydrocephalus, seizures, subdural effusion, or adverse drug effects. For memory retraining, the following are suggested:

1. Establish a consistent daily routine. The patient needs to repeat and rehearse acts.

2. Let the patient respond to questions or commands. Minimize verbal or physical impatience in reaction to the patient's slow, deliberate attempts to respond.

3. Proceed from simple to complex. Break tasks down into component parts. Teach the parts separately and subsequently combine them into a whole.

4. Use multiple sensory modalities to interact with the patient, such as sight, hearing, touch, smell, and movement.

5. Reinforce positively and frequently. Therapeutic sessions should end with "good feelings."

Prosthetic memory aids should be encouraged. In the patient's room, for example, a large clock, calendar, and schedule of daily activities may be hung on the wall. At the bedside, a checklist of common tasks and their component steps may be written or illustrated. Family snapshots or a familiar bedspread may help the patient identify his or her room. The patient may carry a memory book, which lists his or her home address, telephone number, birthdate, and key names.

At some phase of recovery, the **treatment sessions** should ideally occur in a quiet, distraction-free environment. The length of sessions may be only 20–30 minutes in duration. Excessive fatigue or agitation may prompt cancellation or early closure of sessions to avoid an unpleasant or counterproductive experience.

Emotional lability may be managed by distraction techniques, which staff people and family members can be taught in order to deal with unpredictable, disruptive emotional outbursts.

Symptoms of depression may be due to a growing self-awareness of the degree and extent of disability. Depression may lead to suicidal ideation and, in some cases, suicidal gestures. Psychiatric consultation is important **prior to and after discharge.** Suicide precautions may be necessary. The use of antidepressant medication has had varied success.

Impairment in **judgment** and **impulse control** may be met with firm, clear guidance. Attention should focus on residual assets and reasonable goals. Unrealistic expectations should not be nurtured for the sake of "keeping hope alive." Patients should be evaluated on what they have demonstrated, not on what they claim they can do. Climbing ladders, using power tools, driving a car, and other potentially hazardous activities should be prohibited at home until the patient has been satisfactorily evaluated. Patients may often have the physical capability of performing the task but lack the judgment to complete it safely and responsibly.

Unpredictable episodes of **combative** or **highly agitated behavior** may be difficult to manage by time out or isolation rooms alone. There is no clearly established drug of first choice. Propranolol, methylphenidate, thorazine, and haloperidol have had variable trials. Current experience, adverse effects, dosage, and treatment criteria should be understood by the prescribing physician and rehabilitation team.

Social withdrawal may be managed by close family support, frequent opportunity to practice successful social interaction, sound sleep, and a productive daytime schedule. Contact with crowds, overstimulating group activities, intolerant patients on the floor, and unsupportive family behavior should be avoided.

UNILATERAL NEGLECT OF AN EXTREMITY

Patients may neglect an affected upper or lower extremity. Brightly colored labels may be attached to the bedrail, shirt sleeve, or pant leg on the affected side. During an activity, the patient may be positioned so that the unaffected side is closer to the wall of the room and the neglected limb is closer to activity. Descriptive words should be preferred over positional words. For example, an attendant might say, "Hold the fork with your weak hand," rather than "with your left hand." In a sitting position, a lap tray or table may allow the patient's neglected upper extremity to be placed in his or her direct field of vision.

COMMUNICATION

However elementary, a reliable method of communication is essential for the patient's active participation in a rehabilitative program. Depending on the patient's deficits, the speech pathologist can recommend guidelines for people to use in interacting with the patient. Proper and regular evaluations are important in revising these guidelines to take advantage of subtle but significant improvements in expression and comprehension. Augmentative communication devices have provided many nonvocal patients with the ability to communicate with others.

MOTOR INCOORDINATION AND WEAKNESS

Splints, positioning, and passive range of motion exercises (b.i.d.) constitute preventive measures against the development of serious contractures of muscles and joints in the upper and lower extremities.

The progression of mobility depends on the patient's ability to independently perform each major motor activity, such as rolling over in bed, sitting, standing, transferring, walking, climbing steps, and eventually ambulating outdoors. Patients will vary in their eventual means of locomotion.

There are different methods of managing motor incoordination, spasticity, and weakness that are detailed elsewhere in this manual. A physiatrist and physical therapist should be consulted early in the patient's course.

SELF-CARE

Dressing, undressing, grooming, hygiene, toileting, and feeding represent important survival skills for the patient. Resting splints for the upper extremity may provide a more functional position, inhibit abnormal reflexes, and minimize contractures.

Skills may be expanded to involve meal preparation, using a knife, cooking over the stove, and placing an emergency call by telephone. The patient may be taught visual scanning when homonymous hemianopia is present. The side of the body that lacks full sensation may receive special attention through touch, pressure, position, and sight.

A home visit may result in specific recommendations for architectural accessibility, modified furniture, grab bars for the bathroom, and tub benches.

A physiatrist and occupational therapist may be consulted to evaluate and assist in patient management.

SOCIAL ISSUES

The family should be formally oriented, regularly seen, and encouraged to participate in discharge planning with select team members. The family should begin to understand the natural history of patients with head injury, the goals of the program, the guidelines for interacting with the patient, and what their capabilities are for taking care of the patient at home and in the community. The personal needs of the spouse, parent, or sibling deserve open, constructive discussion.

Community agencies, programs, and support groups may play a major role in the patient's successful re-entry into the home, work, school, or community.

For those patients with higher levels of skills, an evaluation for school, employment, and driving may be important prior to discharge.

REFERENCES

Annegers JF, et al: Seizures after head trauma, a population study. Neurology *30*:683, 1980.

Bakay L, Glasauer FE: Head Injury. Boston, Little, Brown, 1980.

Cope DN, and Hall K: Head injury rehabilitation: benefits of early intervention. Arch Phys Med Rehabil *63*:433, 1982.

Jennett B, Teasdale G: Management of Head Injuries. Philadelphia, FA Davis, 1981.

Rosenthal M, Griffith E, Bond MR, Miller JD (eds): Rehabilitation of the Traumatic Brain Injured Adult. Philadelphia, FA Davis, 1982.

Rutherford WH, et al: Sequelae of concussion caused by minor head injuries. Lancet *1*:1, 1977.

37

CEREBRAL PALSY

Cerebral palsy is a nonprogressive movement disability resulting from abnormal development of or injury to the immature brain. It is a recognizable pattern of dysfunctional neurologic development.

Incidence and Prevalence. There are over 900,000 people with cerebral palsy in the United States. Prevalence rates vary widely between 150 and 350 per 100,000 people. Incidence differs from 1.5–6.0 per 1000 live births per year, depending on the demographic and health characteristics of the population.

Etiology. Prenatal (25%) causes are genetic maldevelopment (e.g., X-linked spastic diplegia), teratologic injury (e.g., fetal alcohol syndrome), infectious injury (e.g., congenital rubella), and adverse maternal factors (e.g., toxemia). **Perinatal** (50%) causes are associated with prematurity, trauma, or iatrogenic results. **Postnatal** (5%) causes are due to infection, trauma, or iatrogenic results. Twenty per cent of cases, however, are unknown in etiology.

It is likely that many cases of cerebral palsy are the result of a "cascade" of multiple adverse events.

CLINICAL CLASSIFICATION

Region of Involvement. Hemiplegia, diplegia (lower extremities are involved with only minimally affected upper extremities and without oral deficits), and quadriplegia. Paraplegia, triplegia, and monoplegia occur rarely.

Quality of Tone and Movement. Spasticity, hypotonia, athetosis, chorea, ataxia, dystonia, rigidity.

Characteristic Clinical Patterns. Spastic diplegia is a common sequela of prematurity and is often associated with a few problems. Spastic hemiplegia varies in severity and is often of perinatal or postnatal origin. The upper extremity is usually more involved than the lower extremity. Quadriplegia represents a mixture of tone and movement abnormalities, commonly of severe hypoxic origin. Ataxic cerebral palsy is rare and is occasionally misdiagnosed as ataxia telangiectasia or a posterior fossa tumor. Diffuse hypotonia is frequently associated with mental retardation. It should be differentiated from spinal cord trauma, anterior horn cell disease, neuropathy, and myopathy.

DIAGNOSTIC PRINCIPLES

History and physical examination are invaluable. There are no laboratory tests or other procedures that make the diagnosis. The state of arousal, age, medications, type of cerebral palsy, growth, and development necessitate serial documentation over a long period of time. A pediatrician, child neurologist, pediatric physical or occupational therapist, and other consultants may be desirable in a child's comprehensive evaluation and management.

In general, cerebral palsy can best be recognized by assessing the acquisition of voluntary control over movement as the individual develops. Movement is stereotyped in quality and diminished in quantity at any age.

Cerebral palsy is a recognizable pattern of neuromuscular maldevelopment rather than a disease. It is never sufficient to make a diagnosis of cerebral palsy without inquiring actively into cause. A critical consideration of the possible presence of a progressive neurologic disease should always be undertaken.

Cerebral palsy is only one of several disabilities that can result from an insult or malfunction of the central nervous system. Other disabilities include seizures, mental retardation, sensory deficits, and other manifestations of "static encephalopathy."

Patients may present with mixed findings that elude tidy classification. One examiner's "severe spastic diplegia" may be the next examiner's "mild spastic quadriplegia."

The severity of the motor disability does not predict the severity of associated deficits. Some patients with severe athetoid quadriplegia may have complete preservation of cognitive ability despite total physical incapacitation.

There are a few specific clinical presentations that warrant additional comment. Patients with athetoid quadriplegia due to neonatal hyperbilirubinemia (kernicterus) often have profound bilateral sensorineural hearing loss and paresis of upward gaze masking normal intelligence. The majority of patients with right hemiplegia have significant aphasic language problems that will be more important than their articulation deficit. An occasional patient will have involvement of all four extremities (apparent quadriplegia) but with more severe involvement of the upper extremities or oral mechanisms, or both. The term "double hemiplegia" is used to describe this situation because of the similarity of the findings to the combination of a right and left hemiplegia.

INDEPENDENCE

The individual with cerebral palsy should fulfill his or her maximum potential for independence. Admittedly, this disability fosters physical dependency of the disabled individual. This dependency, however, may be greatly increased by psychologic and social forces. Parents should feel competent if they are to instill the sense of self-worth necessary for their child to become independent.

The physician should explicitly inquire about parental and child sense of self-confidence. Do they have correct information about cerebral palsy, its prognosis and appropriate management? How do the parents and child interact? What is their daily routine? How does the child function at school?

Infantilization, rejection, neglect, and other major conflicts within the family should receive the attention of a mental health worker, who should have some experience with clients disabled by cerebral palsy. The model of mental illness should not be inappropriately applied to a stressed family with a physically disabled child.

Explicit discussions on the importance of independence should begin with parents during infancy and continue throughout life. Medical information should be openly shared. Informed decision-making should be encouraged. The physician may advocate the "least restrictive alternative" consistent with the individual's skills for education, residence, work, and recreation. The disabled person may be referred to a rehabilitative vocational counselor and to lay support groups.

GENERAL HEALTH CARE

Individuals with cerebral palsy have the same health needs as other people. There is no substitute for a thorough history and physical examination.

The physician should complete immunizations, arrange access to satisfactory dental care, monitor weight gain or loss and nutritional intake, perform age-appropriate routine health screening (e.g., blood pressure, Pap smear, glaucoma screen), treat chronic constipation and other effects of immobilization vigorously, manage acne and other adolescent health concerns, and suspect superimposed disease unrelated to the patient's cerebral palsy when new signs and symptoms develop.

COMMUNICATION

The ability to communicate varies from developmentally appropriate to severely impaired. In the evaluation, talk to the patient and decide if the communication is age-appropriate. Gestures, mime, facial expression, eye pointing, and manual signing may be functional substitutes for speech. Hearing should be screened routinely. The physician should maintain eye contact when talking with the individual even if an interpreter or communication device is present.

Encourage parents to keep talking to their child, whose responsiveness may be slowly developing. Trained professionals may stimulate the infant with oral motor problems. Speech and language treatment may be indicated at any age.

The emergence of augmentative communication has introduced an important avenue of learning and interaction for people with cerebral palsy. Word boards, optic devices, electronic voice simulators, or microprocessor computers may be recommended by a consulting speech pathologist or communication disorders specialist.

MOBILITY

During infancy and preschool years, a pediatric physical or occupational therapist may apply current principles of neurophysiologic therapy to improve the patient's gross and fine motor skills. Parents should be taught skills in handling their disabled child.

Joint contractures, orthopedic operations, leg length discrepancy, pelvic obliquity, spinal deformity, and dislocated hips may present in adulthood with low back pain; degenerative joint disease (DJD) of the hips, knees, and feet; chronic pain; and a host of other musculoskeletal symptoms.

It should be remembered that orthopedic surgery may correct fixed bone and joint deformities but should not be expected to "cure" the underlying impairment in abnormal muscle control.

COGNITIVE SKILLS

Motor disability often dominates and disguises intact intellectual ability in individuals with cerebral palsy. Hearing deficits and other potentially treatable problems may be masked. It is true that the majority of children with cerebral palsy fall on the borderline or below normal range on aptitude tests. These scores are often in error as predictors of function in an appropriately designed Individualized Educational Program (IEP).

Other related issues regarding the disabled child are discussed elsewhere in this manual.

SELF-CARE

Cerebral palsy may create real barriers to the child's mastery of a whole gamut of mundane tasks, such as feeding, toileting, bathing, dressing, undressing, and grooming. Adaptive clothing, modified utensils, special equipment, and seating systems may greatly facilitate a child's independent self-care and, simultaneously, decrease his or her dependency on others for assistance. As the patient reaches late adolescence, other survival skills become even more critical for independent living.

OTHER ASSOCIATED PROBLEMS

Seizure disorders occur in half of all individuals with cerebral palsy and are managed no differently from other patients with seizures.

Growth failure can be severe, particularly in patients with severe motor disability. Occasionally, a patient will have overt evidence of diabetes insipidus or other dysfunctions of the hypothalamic-pituitary axis.

Gastroesophageal reflux, esophagitis, and gastritis are commonly seen in cerebral palsy and can usually be treated with alterations in food, positioning, and feeding schedule. Only rarely is a gastrostomy and fundoplication necessary.

The vast majority of people with cerebral palsy can live productive, meaningful lives. Although the disability is permanent, the life span is normal for the vast majority. New or different medical problems should be addressed properly and not glibly considered as unmanageable aspects of cerebral palsy.

REFERENCES

Bleck EE: Orthopaedic Management of Cerebral Palsy. Philadelphia, Saunders, 1979.

Bobath K: A Neurophysiological Basis for the Treatment of Cerebral Palsy. Clinics in Developmental Medicine No. 75. Philadelphia, Lippincott, 1980.

Cohen P, Kohn JG: Followup study of patients with cerebral palsy. West J Med 130:6, 1979.

Drillien CM, Drummond MB: Neurodevelopmental Problems in Early Childhood. London, Blackwell, 1977.

Finnie NR: Handling the Young Cerebral-Palsied Child at Home, 2nd ed. New York, Dutton, 1975.

Halpern D: Therapeutic exercises for cerebral palsy, Chap 13, pp 281–324. In Basmajian JV (ed): Therapeutic Exercise, 3rd ed. Baltimore, Williams & Wilkins, 1978.

Herbst JJ: Gastroesophageal reflux. J Pediatr 98:859, 1981.

Spira R: Management of spasticity in cerebral palsied children by peripheral nerve block with phenol. Develop Med Child Neurol 13:164, 1971.

38

AMYOTROPHIC LATERAL SCLEROSIS

Amyotrophic lateral sclerosis (ALS) is a progressive degenerative disorder of motor neurons in the spinal cord, brainstem, and motor cortex. Upper and lower motor neurons are involved. Extraocular muscles and the sphincters of the anus and bladder are usually not affected. Although pain and paresthesias may occur, objective sensory disturbances are rarely observed. The etiology of the disease is unknown. The only treatment is symptomatic.

Every year in the United States, over 5000 new cases of ALS appear with an incidence of 1.5 per 100,000 people. Given its short natural history, its prevalence is about 10,000 cases. Thus, ALS occurs more frequently than chronic spinal muscular atrophy and all the dystrophic conditions of muscle.

The disease is relentlessly progressive. Plateaus do occur. Death occurs within 2–6 years after onset, usually by aspiration or respiratory failure. The patient who presents initially with weakness, fasciculations, and distal musculature atrophy has a better prognosis than a patient who presents with bulbar or respiratory symptoms. In the latter patient, speech, swallowing, and breathing can be profoundly affected.

MUSCLE WEAKNESS

The specific muscle group, its potential substitution patterns, and the degree of weakness determine the impact of the weakness on the patient's daily activities. Selective exercises may discourage disuse atrophy, strengthen unaffected substituting muscles, and minimize easy fatigability. The patient should not exercise to fatigue, as weakness may be aggravated.

Muscle cramps may occur when exercises or activities are excessive for any set of muscles, even the severely involved. Quinine, diazepam, and phenytoin have been used with limited success.

Imbalance about a joint may predispose the patient to contractures, which can increase the effort required to move the joint in daily activities. Active, assisted, or passive range of motion may be prescribed for the affected joints. Rest orthoses (splints) may be prescribed.

A rare dysfunction of the neuromuscular junction has been described and can aggravate fatigue. Electrodiagnosis can confirm this junctional block. Pyridostigmine may be recommended by the consulting neurologist to improve the patient's strength. It may be taken by the patient in relation to a specific function, such as eating.

Work simplification, energy conservation methods, adaptive equipment, and self-help devices may maximize function significantly.

SPASTICITY

Spasticity may produce discomfort and interfere with mobility and self-care. Although drug therapy has been largely disappointing, baclofen may be prescribed for very bothersome symptoms. The starting dose may be 5 mg t.i.d. and increased to 40–80 mg total daily dosage with clinical titration.

DEPENDENT EDEMA

With the loss of the muscle pump, dependent edema may occur. Provided the patient does not have esophageal reflux or respiratory embarrassment, the feet may be elevated or the foot of the bed raised on blocks. Elevating wheelchair leg rests and gradient support hose may be tried.

DECREASED MOBILITY

With weakening of the dorsiflexors at the ankles, painless foot-drop appears. Gait disturbances become noticeable. After walking stops, mobility continues to deteriorate and there is dependency on attendants for passive locomotion and transfers. Light-weight plastic ankle-foot orthoses can stabilize the ankle for more efficient, safer standing or walking. One or two canes may improve balance and safety. A wheelchair is essential when walking ceases to be independent. For severely disabled patients, a Hoyer lift and a motorized hospital bed can facilitate care greatly and minimize serious back strain among attendants.

DECREASED SELF-CARE

Progressive impairment in dressing, undressing, grooming, hygiene, and toileting parallels the loss of ambulation. Home modifications, adaptive clothing, self-help devices, and special equipment may facilitate self-care in the face of growing demands for assistance.

SWALLOWING DIFFICULTY

Choking, malnutrition, and aspiration are serious complications of ALS, particularly in patients with bulbar symptoms. The patient should eat or be fed from a sitting position. The neck should be flexed, not extended. Patients handle solids better than liquids. Despite these efforts, however, pills may be difficult to swallow whole. Thick, ropy mucus and sialorrhea may aggravate problems related to swallowing.

Pureed food should be avoided. Fresh white bread, peanut butter, and other sticky foodstuffs should be discouraged.

Temperature, taste, and texture stimulating food may "activate" relatively spared musculature. Soft foods that hold together can be swallowed more easily than foods that fall apart (e.g., applesauce). Custards and casseroles may be eaten this way. Similarly, pills may be put in a bite of custard or jelly and thereby swallowed as a bolus.

Chocolate, uncooked milk products, and other mucus-producing items should be avoided. The thick, ropy mucus may be dissolved by placing a papase tablet under the patient's tongue 10 minutes before meals. Alternatively, a small amount of papaya-based meat tenderizer may be swabbed over the tongue just prior to meals.

Sialorrhea responds only briefly, if at all, to anticholinergic medication. Unilateral transtympanic neurectomy and parotid duct ligation may be effective for about 6 months. If sialorrhea persists, the other side may be operated on.

A diminished gag reflex, inadequate food ingestion, and poor fluid intake pose serious threats of malnutrition. For the patient with hand control, intermittent passage of an oral feeding tube may be taught when the gag reflex is decreased. A gastrostomy or cervical esophagostomy may be recommended. The latter procedure permits safe feeding in sitting, minimizes skin irritation or stomatitis, and reduces the risk of peritonitis. Heavy duty electric or portable battery-operated aspirators are beneficial for outpatient use.

RESPIRATORY FAILURE

Restrictive lung impairment, weak respiratory musculature, and obstruction of the upper airway due to atrophic muscles predispose the patient to life-threatening, and often fatal, ventilatory failure. Influenza and pneumococcal vaccinations should be given routinely. Succinylcholine for anesthesia should be avoided because of potentially deleterious hyperkalemia and cardiac arrest. In the final stages of ALS, the patient and family face a decision to use continuous mechanical ventilation as the only means of sustaining life. The decision is highly individual.

SPEECH

Laborious articulation, hypernasality, and a strained voice characterize the speech deficit in ALS. Energy conservation techniques should be taught. Fatigue-producing drills and exercises should be discouraged. Writing and gesturing are satisfactory substitutes for speech. The speech pathologist may recommend a communication board with letters, words, phrases, and pictures or a portable electronic communicator.

PSYCHOSOCIAL ISSUES

Situational or reactive depression is exacerbated with the loss of each functional activity. Death and dying become a real issue with the patient and family. Suicide is rarely encountered. Ideally, a social worker, psychologist, counselor, or mental health professional should discuss psychosocial problems on a regular basis. The effect on the family should be discussed openly. Tranquilizers may aggravate weakness. Antidepressants are usually ineffective.

Local chapters of the Amyotrophic Lateral Sclerosis Foundation and the Muscular Dystrophy Association offer specific patient services and limited coverage for outpatient care.

REFERENCES

DeLisa JA, Mikuclic MA Miller RM, Melnick RR: Amyotrophic lateral sclerosis, comprehensive management. Am Fam Physician 19:137, 1979.

Sivak ED, Gipson WT, Hanson MR: Long-term management of respiratory failure in amyotrophic lateral sclerosis. Ann Neurol 12:18, 1982.

Smith RA, Norris FJ Jr: Symptomatic care of patients with amyotrophic lateral sclerosis. J Am Med Assoc 234:715, 1975.

39

MULTIPLE SCLEROSIS

Multiple sclerosis is a progressive disorder of myelin degeneration affecting the optic nerve, brain, and spinal cord. Its etiology is unknown. In Canada, northern United States, and northern Europe, the incidence is 30–80 per 100,000 per annum, whereas in southern United States and Europe the incidence is 6–14 per 100,000 per annum. The female to male ratio is 2:1. Six out of 10 patients have their initial symptoms between 20 and 40 years. Onset before 15 or after 60 is rare. Gross estimates of prevalence in the United States are more than 400,000, not including people with other demyelinating disorders. Diagnosis often occurs months to years after the initial symptoms. There is no known cure.

Exacerbation and remission characterize the natural course of multiple sclerosis in 9 out of 10 patients. The spectrum of progression, however, varies from symptom-free status for many years to an unrelenting downward course of frequent episodes of exacerbation. One out of 10 patients experiences a steady, unremitting progression.

A relatively more favorable prognosis is associated with a number of clinical variables: The onset is before 35 years; is precipitous; is followed by resolution of symptoms within a month; involves only optic neuritis, sensory (nonmotor), or noncerebellar signs; and is without Babinski sign. Total remissions or well-defined exacerbations of less than 2 months are favorable indicators. The patient who walks at initial assessment or who has mild cerebellar and pyramidal signs at 5 years postonset tends to have a less disabling course. For any given patient, however, precise prognostication is unobtainable.

REHABILITATIVE MANAGEMENT

The disabling manifestations of multiple sclerosis may include the following: easy fatigability, weakness, spasticity, motor incoordination, ataxia, tremors, visual loss, diplopia, dysarthria, urinary incontinence, and paresthesias. Psychosocial symptoms range from profound depression to unrealistic optimism. Prolonged immobilization, contractures, falls, and social embarrassment from incontinence create other problems for the patient. Blindness, mobility by wheelchair, assisted self-care, frequent exacerbations, and movement disorders obviously have serious consequences for the person's ability to work and live independently.

ACTH has been used to shorten or blunt severe exacerbations. Some patients definitely respond to ACTH, but there is no apparent long-term benefit.

Strategies to deal with these various symptoms are discussed elsewhere in this manual. Multidisciplinary clinics and consumer-oriented programs are accessible to many more people with multiple sclerosis.

REFERENCES

Kraft GH, Freal JE, Coryell JK, et al: Multiple sclerosis: early prognostic guidelines. Arch Phys Med Rehabil 62:54, 1981.

Multiple sclerosis. (Special issue) Physiotherapy 68:144, 1982.

Treatment of multiple sclerosis and comprehensive long-term care for multiple sclerosis patients. (Special issue) Neurol 39:8, 1980.

40

PARKINSON'S DISEASE

Parkinson's disease is a slowly progressive disorder of movement. Its onset is usually between 50 and 60 years. In the United States, the incidence is 20 per 100,000 people per annum with a prevalence of 100–150 per 100,000 general population. Sixty percent of patients are males. In general, 5–10 years following onset of symptoms, Parkinson's disease is moderately disabling. Mortality rates are three times those of the general population owing to infections, falls, trauma, and other complications of immobility. Nearly 90% of cases are idiopathic in origin.

STAGES OF DISABILITY

Five stages of disability and symptoms characterize the course of Parkinson's disease. In *Stage I,* mild resting tremor, rigidity, bradykinesia, dysarthria, trunk tilt, fine motor incoordination, and facial immobility are noticeable but not disabling. Symptoms often present in a unilateral or hemiparetic fashion.

Stage II is mildly disabling as symptoms appear bilaterally and standing posture becomes stooped. Gait is a shuffle. Fatigue, bradykinesia, and weakness impair home and work activities. The wrists assume a slightly dorsiflexed position. The flexed metacarpophalangeal and distal and extended proximal interphalangeal joints characterize the hand deformity. The pattern of truncal and limb contracture is noted.

In *Stage III,* moderate disability involves a festinating gait. Retropulsion initially and propulsion later interfere with stopping, starting, turning, and stepping backward. Self-care activities are tediously performed and often require attendant help. Falls become a real threat to the patient's safety. The PIP joints of the hands become hyperextended as the DIP joints and wrist become more flexed. With an ankle in slight varus, hammertoes (2nd to 5th) and a hyperextended big toe characterize the striatal foot. Leg cramps, tight ankles, and skin breakdown over the toes may be partly remediated by firm, supportive shoes with a large toe box.

In *Stage IV,* marked rigidity, akinesia, and poor standing balance are severely disabling, as in fine motor incoordination. Thus, safe, independent ambulation is confined to the home at best and self-care skills require assistance. Contractures are increasingly more refractory to conventional stretching exercises. Tremor, interestingly, is less pronounced.

Stage V represents complete dependency and serious worsening of all preceding patterns of musculoskeletal disability. Aspiration pneumonitis, weight loss, malnutrition, dehydration, and fecal impaction often necessitate a gastrostomy or nasogastric feeding tube. Many patients do not reach this grave level of disability owing to fatal complications in earlier stages.

OTHER COMPLICATIONS

Autonomic dysfunction occurs in varying degrees of severity and may be as disabling as associated movement deficits. Drooling due to excessive salivation, dysphagia from incoordinated hypopharyngeal muscles, delayed emptying of gastric contents, constipation from hypomotile bowels, urinary hesittancy from a neurogenic bladder, syncope from orthostatic hypotension, and excessive perspiration may be present. Horner's syndrome, seborrheic dermatitis, abnormal peripheral sensation of cold or burning, vague aches of muscle and joints, and poor fluid intake may also characterize the patient. Dementia and depression may also occur as a debilitating complication. Each of these complications may compound the musculoskeletal disability and suggest specific rehabilitative strategies described elsewhere in this manual.

MEDICATION

A discussion of drug management is beyond the scope of this section. In principle, drug treatment does not affect the underlying pathologic process but does delay the onset of complications. Medication should be prescribed when symptoms are troublesome, starting with antimuscarinics or amantadine. Levodopa should be employed judiciously because it appears to be effective for only a 3- to 5-year period for the 9 out of 10 patients who are initially prescribed the drug.

A loss in function from a new or different symptom may be due to the adverse effect of a prescribed therapeutic drug. Adverse drug effects can include dyskinetic movement, memory loss, insomnia, confusion, hallucination, paranoid ideation, nightmares, and irritability. Dry mouth, nausea, vomiting, stomach ache, constipation, and anorexia may occur. Hypotension, cardiac arrhythmia, urinary retention, ankle edema, and glaucoma have also been observed with various drugs. Proper drug management is critical in Parkinson's disease.

DRUG HOLIDAY

The beneficial effect of levodopa may be restored or prolonged by a 5- to 7-day drug abstinence in a hospital. In addition, on-off reactions may be curtailed. Most drug holidays involve comprehensive rehabilitative evaluation and teaching.

REHABILITATIVE MANAGEMENT

Because the level of a person's function may change frequently throughout the day, reliance on energy-conserving techniques, attendant help, and adaptive equipment can vary for an individual in a less than predictable fashion. Anticipatory guidance, health education, and attention to psychosocial issues are as important in this condition as in all other disabilities.

The maintenance of safe, independent ambulation depends on the patient's posture, balance, and coordinated movement in starting and stopping. The American Parkinson Disease Association (APDA) suggests the following practical guidelines:*

When walking or standing, the feet should be spread apart about 25 cm (10 in.) and should **not** cross. Feet should lift in an exaggerated manner to discourage shuffling and scuffing. Toes should clear the ground to avoid tripping. Similarly, normal arm swing should be exaggerated. The patient should look ahead, not at the ground. Steps should tend to be longer. In turning, the patient should plan to take a large arc without crossing the feet and always in a forward direction. When the patient realizes that walking is rapid in a forward or backward direction, standing should be promptly assumed. Walking may resume with high, long steps. Talking may be discouraged during ambulation because of its potentially distracting effect on the patient's concentration to walk properly.

Practice may be aided by counting aloud a cadence, marching to music, checking posture in a mirror, walking over deliberately placed, low-lying objects on the floor, or holding objects (e.g., rolled-up magazines, weights) to create a pendulum effect in arm swinging. A firm, comfortable pair of shoes may provide greater stability, compensate for tight ankles, and accommodate hammertoes.

For self-care, clothing may be modified by Velcro closures and zippers. Raised toilet seats, hand rails, grab bars, and large handles or knobs may be recommended. Prolonged sitting or bed lying should be avoided.

Dysarthric speech may be helped by exercises in deep breathing, rhythm, and articulation taught by a speech pathologist, who may also be consulted for drooling and dysphagia.

---

*Lavigne J: Home Exercises for Patients with Parkinson's Disease, pp 13–14. New York, APDA.

HOME PROGRAM

A conscientious program of home exercises should be recommended by the physician and taught by a physical or occupational therapist. Because of the fluctuation in overall strength, endurance, and coordination, the patient is frequently faced with a return to higher levels of physical activity following prolonged periods of immobilization. The patient should **gradually** increase the quantity of discrete exercises and take frequent rest pauses during general physical activity. Overexertion, stumbling, and discomfort should signal cessation or truncation of the exercise schedule. The APDA has suggested a home program of muscle conditioning, contracture prevention, and improved coordination. It is advisable to have a physical or occupational therapist assist a patient in developing an individual home program and, if necessary, make a home visit for adaptive equipment and architectural barriers.

REFERENCES

Duvoisin R: Parkinsonism. Clinical Symposia (CIBA) 28:1, 1976.
Weiner WJ, Roller WC, et al: Drug holidays and management of Parkinson's disease. Neurol 30:1257, 1980.

41

ARTHRITIS

Symptomatic arthritis affects nearly 10–12% of the general population. One fourth of cases are due to rheumatoid arthritis and the vast majority result from degenerative joint disease (DJD) or osteoarthritis. Over a million Americans between 35 and 50 years of age are disabled by rheumatoid arthritis.

Although the term "arthritis" implies a primary role for inflammation, this discussion applies to all chronic disorders that cause joint pain, destruction, or dysfunction. Whether arthritis affects the peripheral joints or the spine, the same basic principles apply. Tailoring the program to the individual patient demands only that certain distinctions be made. Single or multiple joints may be acutely, subacutely, or chronically inflamed.

(The reader should refer to the index for other discussions regarding arthritis.)

FUNCTIONAL PROBLEMS AND EVALUATION

Functional limitations of arthritis result from the following: pain due to inflammation or loss of cartilage; joint deformity; weakness due to disuse atrophy or pain inhibition; loss of motion from an effusion, joint surface incongruity, or joint capsule contracture; and joint instability due to ligamentous laxity and muscle atrophy.

EVALUATION

The evaluation begins with an assessment of the number, location, and severity of the affected joints. The presence or absence of the following should be noted: inflammation; effusion; limitation in joint range; muscle weakness or atrophy; deformity or abnormal posture; and functional limitations of ambulation or self-care.

MANAGEMENT

The **goals** of management are to maintain comfort, preserve function, and prevent deformities. The application of modalities, joint range of motion, strengthening exercises, orthotics, preventive protection of joints, walking aids, adaptive equipment, and health education constitute important strategies.

PHYSICAL MODALITIES

Superficial heat provides relief from pain by inhibiting the conduction of pain impulses in nerve fibers, by reflex relaxation of muscle spasm, and by the reduction of stiffness.

Hot baths or **showers** are most practical for home use, especially for the treatment of generalized morning stiffness.

Paraffin baths can be done at home and, although messy, provide an excellent heat source to hands before range of motion exercises.

Hot packs are useful in a clinic or office setting for specific joints before exercise. A heating pad should be used cautiously to avoid burns and can be used at home.

Heat lamps provide a source of localized heat for specific joints or, if used in combination, for larger areas.

Deep heat is applied by ultrasound and effectively heats the joint capsule and surrounding ligaments. This modality is contraindicated in acutely inflamed joints. In its most effective application, it facilitates range of motion exercises for joint contracture by increasing collagen distensibility.

Cold application has the advantage of deeper penetration and longer duration of pain relief. It is not contraindicated in acute inflammatory conditions. A major disadvantage is its failure to relieve stiffness.

RANGE OF MOTION EXERCISES

These exercises should be performed daily. Ideally, the exercises should follow the application of superficial heat, which has decreased pain and muscle spasm. Each involved joint should be ranged to its maximum at least once a day. In acutely inflamed joints, two to three near-maximal ranges should be followed by one maximal range for each joint. A more vigorous regimen may aggravate pain, inflammation, and muscle spasm. As a rule, an exercise program should **not** produce pain that lasts for more than 30–60 minutes.

Active ranging is preferable if the joint pain is not so great as to prevent the patient from completing full range of motion.

Active assisted ranging is indicated if the patient is unable to complete full range of motion actively. When the patient moves the joint within the limits of pain tolerance, the patient is better able to maintain muscle strength and to encourage the afferent input from the muscles that control the joint.

An **overhead pulley** may help a patient to maintain a suitable home program of ranging affected shoulders. **Chest expansion** and **spinal extension** exercises are indicated in patients with ankylosing spondylitis. **Daily proning** (lying prone) may help to prevent or minimize hip and knee flexion contractures. For joints that are contracted, the use of prolonged passive stretch and, if not contraindicated, ultrasound for deep heat is more effective than range of motion exercises alone.

MUSCLE STRENGTHENING EXERCISES

Isotonic exercises involve joint motion and can increase pain and inflammation. Nevertheless, progressive resistive exercises may be tolerated in patients with nonacute arthritis. The range of motion may be arbitrarily restricted. Thus, progressive resistive exercises may be performed in comfort without a loss of therapeutic efficacy.

Isometric exercise is maximal muscle contraction with joint immobility. Many patients tolerate isometric better than isotonic exercises. For maintenance, only one to two maximal contractions per day for each muscle group is necessary. A simple home maintenance program of isometric exercises may utilize a beach ball or large rubber bands to provide continuous resistance during exercises.

ORTHOTICS

Orthoses (braces, splints) can immobilize joints and may effectively reduce pain, muscle spasm, and inflammation. **Rest splints** may be worn during sleep, naps, and other periods of relative inactivity. During intense inflammation, they may be worn during the daytime. The development of deformities may be minimized by rest splints. The wrist, hands, and knees are common sites for immobilization.

Functional orthoses are worn during activity mainly to protect inflamed joints. Presumably, pain decreases and function improves. A functional splint for the wrist orthoses can be made of plastic, leather, or cloth. The cervical collar and small ring splints for the digits are other examples.

Dynamic orthoses vary in efficacy. For example, the effectiveness of an orthosis to control ulnar deviation but allow hand function is disputed by some physicians.

PREVENTIVE PROTECTION OF JOINTS

Customary activities of daily life include movements that stress inflamed joints and often lead to deformities. This is particularly true in the hands, where force of grasp translates into forces along the tendons, which favor subluxation and ulnar deviation at the metacarpal-phalangeal joints.

In general, the patient should respect discomfort and, in particular, pain, and strive toward a balance between activity and work. To complete a task, the effort should be minimal and efficient.

Deforming positions should be avoided. The more unstable, weaker, and smaller joints should be used minimally; conversely, the more stable, stronger, and larger joints should be activated more frequently. Each joint should be used in maximum function and anatomic stability. Protracted use of a joint, such as grasping or pushing, should be avoided. The patient should consider only physical activity that he or she can promptly cease if painful symptoms appear. A program of muscle strengthening and contracture prevention should be faithfully maintained. Adaptive equipment and orthoses should be used or worn if they help the patient protect joints.

OTHER INTERVENTIONS

Walking aids may support continued ambulation for patients who can no longer bear weight. Forearm crutches, platform crutches, or modified walkers may effectively unload the multiply involved weight-bearing joints.

A **powered wheelchair or cart** may restore the patient's independent, safe, functional locomotion after bipedal ambulation has ceased or is limited to short indoor distances.

Self-care may be facilitated by self-help devices, adaptive clothing, and modified equipment, such as long handled combs and a raised toilet seat.

Special **shoes** may be extra wide and extra deep to accommodate toe deformities. Metatarsal pads and bars, for example, may be made of polyethylene (Plastazote) and relieve pressure over the metatarsal heads.

Adequate rest is critical for **all** patients with significant arthritis. Patients should learn to balance physical and resting activities, to avoid excessive fatigue, and to restrict use of painfully inflamed joints.

Reconstructive orthopedic surgery may be recommended in selective cases. A discussion of joint prostheses is beyond the scope of this discussion.

REFERENCES

Ehrlich GE (ed): Rehabilitation Management of Rheumatic Conditions. Baltimore, Williams & Wilkins, 1980.

Flatt AE: Care of the Arthritic Hand. St Louis, Mosby, 1983.

Licht S: Arthritis and Physical Medicine. New Haven, Elizabeth Licht, 1969.

Self-Help Manual for Arthritis Patients, The Arthritis Foundation, 1212 Avenue of the Americas, New York, New York 10036

Swezey RL: Arthritis, Rational Therapy and Rehabilitation. Philadelphia, Saunders, 1978.

42

CHRONIC PAIN SYNDROMES

LOW BACK PAIN

The most frequent cause of acute low back pain is acute muscular strain. Chronic low back pain most often involves predisposing contractured or deconditioned musculature. Obesity and weak abdominal musculature may contribute to inadequate intra-abdominal pressure important for full lumbar support. Tight or contractured hip flexor, lumbar paraspinal, and hamstring musculature may increase lumbar lordosis or limit smooth lumbar movement or both.

Radiculopathy, degenerative disc disease, arthritides, neoplasms, compression fracture, spondylolisthesis, and infection can cause acute or chronic low back pain.

Diseases of retroperitoneal and pelvic organs present with a variety of symptoms among which is low back discomfort.

Hysterical low back pain is unusual. More commonly a patient's symptoms may be exaggerated or exacerbated by a low pain threshold, secondary gain, or personality makeup.

Evaluation

History

Acute lumbar strains and radiculopathies are often causally tied to a specific accident or activity. Pain and morning stiffness suggest an arthritic cause. Reflex muscle spasm in the buttocks and hamstring musculature implicate strain. In classic radiculopathy, the discomfort truly radiates into the leg(s) and is exacerbated by prolonged sitting or Valsalva maneuvers. In malignancies, other ominous symptoms are often present and the patient may present with waking up at night from a low back pain. A severe lesion may produce stool or urinary incontinence, paresthesias, and weakness (e.g., ankle twisting, toe dragging).

A detailed history of activity at work, home, and recreation may elucidate the etiology of the low back pain. Family history may reveal an arthritic disorder or, possibly, learned behavior from other similarly disabled people in the home.

A history of **surgery, medication,** and **medical treatment** is critical and may suggest operant pain behavior. Drug abuse may be present.

Physical Examination

A careful and systematic examination of the patient is essential. For a detailed description of a proper evaluation, the reader is referred to a standard textbook or manual on musculoskeletal examination of the low back. The following are guidelines to consider:

A. Inspect and palpate the spine, musculature of the paraspinal and abdominal regions, pelvis, and femur. Look for spinal deformity, pelvic obliquity, spasms, and myofascial trigger points.

B. Instruct the standing patient to keep the knees extended and next flex, extend, bend, and rotate at the lumbar spine. Observe for jerky, dysrhythmic movement.

C. Check out each spinal segment as represented by the respective dermatomes and innervated muscles. Loss of acuity to pin prick and muscle weakness suggest a nerve root lesion.

D. Superficial cutaneous and deep tendon reflexes screen the integrity of the afferent-efferent loop at the spinal cord level. The bulbocavernosus, anal, cremasteric, abdominal, or Babinski reflexes may be performed with the knee and ankle tendon percussions.

E. There are several maneuvers to stress the sacroiliac joint (pelvic compression test, Patrick's test or fabere sign, or Gaenslen's sign); hip joint (Patrick's test or fabere sign); spinal cord, cauda equina, or sciatic nerve (straight leg raising test, cross leg straight raising test, Hoover's sign, Kernig's sign); intervertebral disc (Naffziger's test, Milgram's test, or valsalva).

F. Measure the thigh and calf circumferences. A level 10 cm below and 20 cm above the fibular head may be routinely adopted.

G. Measure for true leg length discrepancy, using the anterior superior iliac spine and the apex of the medial malleolus. Break up the measurement at the medial joint line of the knee in the presence of a knee flexion contracture.

H. Observe the patient during sitting, standing, walking, lying, climbing steps, and other activities.

I. Check the joint range of motion at the hips, knees, and ankles.

J. Check for consistency. Attempt to isolate the pathologic anatomy. Rule out malingering, hysteria, and conversion reaction.

Laboratory and Radiology

Laboratory and radiologic procedures should be individualized for each patient. An otherwise healthy person, for example, with a clear history of acute low back strain and absent neurologic deficits may be treated symptomatically **without** further diagnostic procedures. If the patient fails to respond within 10–14 days, investigation may proceed.

Blood or urinary tests are seldom useful for most patients with low back pain. If a rheumatologic disorder is considered, antinuclear antibody, rheumatoid factor, HLA-B27, and sedimentation rate may be ordered. Depending on the suspected osteopenic condition, a serum calcium, phosphorus, and alkaline phosphatase may be recommended.

Electromyography and nerve conduction studies may be extremely useful and provide objective evidence of pathology. When a dysfunction of the primary motor unit is suspected, electrodiagnostic studies should be ordered as a first line procedure. The screen may be consistent with a compression of a nerve root(s). The precise level of the herniating disc, however, cannot be diagnosed with any great deal of certainty.

Plain radiograph, AP and lateral, may reveal degenerative joint disease (DJD), spondylolysis, congenital bony abnormalities, malignant bony lesions, compression fractures, and extravertebral lesions. Pseudoarthrosis or slipped instruments may be detected in a patient with previous spine fusion and instrumentation.

Bone scan may be indicated to rule out infection or bony inflammation in DJD and spondylolisthesis.

Computerized tomography may be quite sensitive in identifying disc herniation, spinal stenosis, and occult malignancies.

Myelogram may be indicated in the evaluation.

Acute Management

Rest is the cornerstone of management for acute low back pain. At home, the patient should lie on a firm mattress. A 5/8- or 3/4-inch thick sheet of plywood may be sandwiched between the box spring and mattress, especially underlying the trunk and lower extremities of the patients. In the hospital, a semi-Fowler's bed position may be more effective in relieving muscle spasm. Clinical evaluation and judgment determine the recommended amount of strict rest, limited physical activities, and return to work.

Muscle relaxants may be prescribed for the first 7–10 days to relieve reflex muscle spasm. Cyclobenzaprine (Flexeril) 10 mg P.O. t.i.d.–q.i.d. may be prescribed. Adverse reactions may include drowsiness, dry mouth, dizziness, fatigue, nausea, constipation, and many others. Cyclobenzaprine should not be prescribed with MAO inhibitors or tricyclic antidepressants. Confusion, agitation, hyperpyrexia, and muscle rigidity may signal overdosage. Diazepam 5 mg P.O. t.i.d.–q.i.d. is effective but potentially an abused substance.

Analgesics may be desirable. An injectable analgesic may be recommended for the first 2–3 days in a patient who is hospitalized. Further need for narcotic analgesia should be prescribed on a **time-contingent basis**, not "p.r.n." Operant pain or drug-seeking behavior should be discouraged.

Heat modalities may effectively relieve acute pain and promote muscle relaxation. Deep heat (short-wave or microwave diathermy) can cover a large area, although some patients prefer superficial heat through hot packs. Ultrasound cannot be efficiently applied over the broad, large area of the back and, theoretically, may aggravate mechanical nerve root compression by increasing the inflammatory response.

Massage may "break up" myofascial trigger points and muscle spasm. A specific technique may be taught to a spouse, friend, or family member.

Therapeutic exercises may begin with isometric strengthening exercises of the four extremities. When muscle spasm and pain have subsided considerably within 2–3 days of strain, isometric exercises of the abdominal and gluteal musculature may be recommended. If the patient remains stable or improves, **pelvic tilt** exercises may be taught within 1–2 days.

Toward the end of the week, the physical therapist may be requested to teach more advanced exercises that strengthen the flexor muscles of the lumbosacral spine and that stretch the extensors of the back. These **daily** performed exercises are popularly referred to as **William's flexion exercises.** In general, it is unsatisfactory to hand a patient a sheet of the exercises **without** one or more teaching sessions by a physical therapist.

The exercises include pelvic tilt and abdominal-gluteal sets; head-shoulder curls; knee-chest; trunk flexion; hamstring stretch: thigh-hip stretch; and wall back-flattening.

Contraindicated are double leg raises and sit-ups.

Aggressive, imprudent prescription for exercises may aggravate symptoms and possibly exacerbate the underlying problem. For example, an increase in symptoms within 2 or more hours following the cessation of exercise suggests increased disc pressure and nerve root irritation. In this situation, exercises should be temporarily discontinued or modified.

Except in conditions that require bed rest, encourage the patient to maintain activity within pain tolerance. If possible, have the patient return to work with recommended restrictions. Where and when appropriate, this is usually preferred over keeping the patient out of work.

Limit medications to the first 1–2 weeks during the acute stages. In that period, patients will derive the most benefit from analgesics and muscle relaxants. Long-term anti-inflammatory medications, however, may be indicated in a patient with underlying inflammatory bone disease.

Obesity is a major aggravating factor. Particularly in the patient who develops chronic or recurrent back pain, weight loss and control constitute a major part of management.

Suspect a strong component of psychosocial overlay in a patient who has the following course:

1. After 3–4 weeks, the patient continues to prefer to stay off work and to let others in the household perform daily chores.

2. Patient seeks more medication, surgery, or testing in excess of what the physician considers reasonable.

3. Patient tends to comply poorly to recommendations.

A clinical psychologist or psychiatrist with rehabilitation experience should be consulted. As part of the evaluation, a Minnesota Multiphasic Personality Inventory (MMPI) may be recommended.

Chronic Low Back Pain

When the low back pain persists for 6 months or more or is a recurrent problem or both, the patient may be a candidate for a comprehensive evaluation at a pain clinic. Baseline evaluation may include the following: detailed history and complete physical examination; pain diary kept by the patient for 2–4 weeks; diagnostic testing; assessment of mobility (by physical therapist); assessment of self-care (by occupational therapist); vocational evaluation (by vocational counselor); psychologic interview and testing (by psychologist or psychiatrist); social evaluation (by social worker); and final multidisciplinary conference to determine the patient's eligibility for an inpatient or outpatient pain program. A physiatrist, neurologist, neurosurgeon, orthopedist, and anesthesiologist usually constitute the other participating physicians.

Special Causes of Low Back Pain

Radiculopathy

Radiating symptoms and paresthesias strongly suggest a radiculopathy. In severe cases, specific muscle weakness, fecal soiling, or bladder dysfunction may be present. Neurologic and musculoskeletal examination may yield positive signs of radiculopathy. **Electrodiagnosis** and computerized tomography may identify the defects. Myelography may be performed selectively in nonoperative patients or as a mandatory preoperative test to determine the surgical site.

Strict bed rest is the key to successful management. The patient may assume a semi-Fowler's position, which is usually the most comfortable for the patient. Pelvic traction at 30–40 lb may be added. The pull should promote flattening of the lumbar lordosis, not increase it. Traction probably insures that the patient complies with strict bed rest orders rather than altering the site of pathology significantly. Hanging traction utilizes the patient's body weight and may be preferred over pelvic traction alone.

Reflex muscle spasm may be managed by heat, massage, and muscle relaxants. Some physicians have injected steroid medication epidurally in severe cases.

The use of **chemonucleolysis** is controversial as an alternative to surgery. It is **not** indicated in the following situations: normal discogram; total block by myelogram; vague diagnosis; tumor; cauda equina syndrome; spinal stenosis; and rapidly progressive loss of motor, bladder, and bowel function. Allergy to the chymopapain and previous injections are other contraindications.

In the presence of neurologic deterioration, progressive bowel or bladder symptoms, or intractable pain following a 2-week period of conservative management, **surgery** should be evaluated. Fortunately, the vast majority of patients respond to conservative therapy. Conversely, past experience suggests that surgery is not the panacea to low back pain. The patient with high hypochondriasis, depression, and hysteria on an MMPI, for example, is at high risk for recurrent symptoms following surgery.

Spondylolisthesis

A spondylolytic defect in the pars interarticularis (oblique plain radiographs) and spondylolisthesis (lateral radiograph) may be found in an physically active adolescent or young adult with chronic low back pain. The sliding of one vertebra over another may be graded according to the percentage of body overlap: Grade I, 25%; II, 50%; III, 75%; and IV, 100%.

Surgical consultation should be sought for a patient with Grade III or IV spondylolisthesis. Lumbar flexion, hamstring stretch, and abdominal strengthening should be recommended for patients with Grade I or II in order to discourage further angulation between L5 and S1 vertebrae. The amount of shear between them may be minimized by the exercises that decrease the lumbar lordosis. Back extension can increase this shear force at L5 and S1 and aggravate symptoms and thus should be avoided.

The patient should have a bone scan. If the scan is positive, a patient with a milder case of spondylolisthesis may wear a brace that limits extension but allows flexion. In more severe cases, the brace should be a lumbosacral support with metal stays or other rigid braces. These patients should wear a brace for 2–3 months before exercises begin.

Degenerative Spondylosis

Nerve root involvement should be ruled out. A bone scan may identify the level of bony inflammatory response. Long-term anti-inflammatory medication may be recommended. Acute flare-ups should be treated with heat and muscle relaxants. Within the patient's pain tolerance, an exercise program for home should be recommended and consist of lumbar flexion and hamstring stretch.

Compression Fractures

Compression fractures occur most frequently in patients with osteoporosis. Specific causes of abnormal bone metabolism should be ruled out. Neural involvement should be looked for in careful history and examination.

Fractures may be diagnosed by plain radiographs and bone scans of the spine. Scans may be positive early in the course when plain radiographs may be negative. As many as 7–10 days may lapse before clear radiographic evidence is appreciated. Bone scans are useful to rule out metastatic disease. Serum calcium, phosphorus, alkaline phosphatase, and immunoelectrophoresis may be recommended.

In the acute phase, bed rest and analgesics should be suggested for a 10- to 14-day period. Following this rest, the patient may be braced in **extension,** not flexion. The level of compression fracture(s) will determine the precise type of bracing. A lower lumbar level requires a lumbosacral corset. A Taylor or Florida-type brace with shoulder straps incorporates the thorax and pulls the shoulders into extension in patients with high lumbar or low thoracic lesions. An orthopedic surgeon, physiatrist, or orthotist should be consulted if the type of brace is in question.

Back extension and full proning exercises should be taught for home therapy 2–3 times a day. A physical therapist and occupational therapist should participate in the evaluation, teaching, and monitoring of the patient.

Sacroiliac Sprain and Inflammation

The sacroiliac joint is difficult to treat. For **sprain,** bed rest, nonsteroidal anti-inflammatory drugs, and analgesics may be sufficient. A trochanteric cinch may provide some relief and is a 4- to 5-cm wide webbing belt that is cinched tightly around the hips between the greater trochanter and iliac crest.

For **ankylosing spondylitis,** the relentless but variable progression of hip flexion, thoracolumbar kyphosis, and cervical flexion may be retarded by vigorous spine extension exercises, nonsteroidal anti-inflammatory medication, and proper posture. Spine surgery and total hip replacement may be indicated. A rheumatologist should be consulted for medical management.

REFERENCES

Calliet R: Low Back Syndromes. Philadelphia, Davis, 1981.
Freeman C, Carsyn D, Louks J: The use of MMPI with low back pain patients. J Clin Psychol 32:294, 1976.
Friedmann LW: Exercises to keep low back pain away. Patient Care, February 1977, pp 91–130.
Jensen GM: Biomechanics of the lumbar intervertebral disk, a review. Phys Ther 60:765, 1980.
MacNab I: Backache. Baltimore, Williams & Wilkins, 1977.
Mennel JMcM: Back Pain. Boston, Little, Brown, 1960.
Rothman RH, Simeone FA: The Spine, 2nd ed., Vols I and II. Philadelphia, Saunders, 1982.

SHOULDER PAIN

Shoulder-hand syndrome, adhesive capsulitis, and rotator cuff rupture are a few major problems of physical shoulder disability.

Mobilization and pain control are two shared goals of these conditions. Some aspects of shoulder disability in cerebrovascular accidents (CVAs) are discussed elsewhere in this manual (Chapter 35).

Shoulder-Hand Syndrome

Shoulder-hand syndrome has been called reflex sympathetic dystrophy, Sudeck's atrophy, causalgia, and reflex neurovascular syndrome of the upper extremity. This chronic disability is characterized by pain, edema, atrophy, dystrophic skin, and restrictive joint range of the shoulder and hand. About 10% of cases involve both sides.

The etiology and pathophysiology of shoulder-hand syndrome are unknown. Venous and lymphatic drainage of the hand and arm are located primarily on the dorsal surface. Drainage depends on the muscle pump of the hand, wrist, and shoulder and, probably, on repeated elevation of the arm. Noxious stimuli to the upper extremity can decrease motion and impair the muscle pump, resulting in edema formation and aggravation of painful symptoms.

Another theory suggests that afferent stimuli from an injury to the arm, shoulder, or chest travel to the spinal cord and enter the sympathetic pathways via the internuncial neuron pool. The effect is massive vasomotor instability, edema, and perpetuation of pain. The inciting source of noxious stimuli is aggravated and results in a reverberating circuit.

Conditions Associated with Syndrome

Trauma accounts for nearly 40–50% of cases. Fracture, for example, to the wrist, hand, elbow, and forearm has been associated with the syndrome. Other conditions include CVA and hemiplegia, postmyocardial infarction, chest or cardiac surgery, neuropathy, and DJD and arthritis. The syndrome can be idiopathic. Hysteria, hypochondriasis, and a "lack of motivation" do not produce the signs of this syndrome.

Stages of Development

Stage 1. The dorsa of the hand and wrist swell and lose the fine wrinkles over the interphalangeal joints. Voluntary or passive flexion of the wrist and fingers is painful and limited in motion. The hand is tender. The elbow joint is usually spared. Similarly, the shoulder may be painful with limited rotation and abduction. The skin of the hand may be moist, pale, cool, and hypersensitive to touch.

Stage 2. Pain may begin to decrease in the shoulder and hand. Edema may begin to subside in the hand and wrist. Skin and nails become atrophic. Restricted joint range may persist in the shoulder, wrist, and fingers. Plain anterior-posterior radiograph of the hand may reveal a characteristic moth-eaten, patchy, spotty osteoporosis of the hand bones.

Stage 3. Atrophy of the skin and muscles may continue with further and often irreversible loss of joint range and function. The hand may assume a clawlike appearance and paradoxically feel painless and nontender at this stage. This may occur within 6–12 months of symptom onset.

Management

Treatment—joint range of motion, superficial heat, deep heat, medication, and sympathetic block—is aimed at three objectives: **reduce pain, control edema,** and **improve joint range**. The goal is restoration or improvement in function.

A. **Analgesics** may provide sufficient relief to allow treatment and encourage more spontaneous use of the limb. Salicylates 300–500 mg P.O. q4–6 hours may be prescribed within the limits of their general adverse effects. Codeine may be necessary 30–60 minutes prior to active therapy, particularly during the first 7–10 days. Avoid narcotics over any prolonged period.

B. **Steroids** have been regarded as helpful by some physicians. Triamcinolone diacetate 16 mg P.O. q6 hours for 14–21 days has been recommended. It is available in 1-, 2-, 4-, 8-, and 16-mg tablets (Aristocort). The dose should be tapered over a 7- to 8-day period. Other physicians have recommended equivalent or smaller doses of prednisone 20–60 mg daily over 14 days and tapering according to the response.

C. **Physical modalities** may reduce pain and edema. Paraffin dips are particularly useful for clinic or home therapy. Contrast baths also require hand immersion and can be applied under supervision. Hot packs, ice packs, massage, and deep heat by ultrasound can also be utilized. During or immediately following deep heat, the tight shoulder capsule should be stretched. Depending on the modality, a b.i.d.–q.i.d. program may be set up between clinic and home.

D. **Edema control** can be done by wrapping the swollen fingers individually with elastic twine (distal to proximal direction), wrapping the arm with an elastic bandage, or wearing a custom-fitted elastic glove. Pillows can be placed under an elevated arm. More effectively, the arm can be wrapped in an Ace bandage and hung by an overhanging sling. The hand should be elevated above the level of the patient's heart. This sling may be used during the day and night. A Jobst pump or other intermittent pneumatic devices may be tried to reduce swelling in the wrist and hand.

E. **Therapeutic exercise** consists of active and passive range of motion t.i.d.–q.i.d., usually in conjunction with physical modalities. The goal is full shoulder abduction and external rotation. Exercises should retard disuse atrophy of muscles and contribute to greater joint range of motion. Reckless painful passive stretch should be avoided. Analgesics or transcutaneous electrical nerve stimulation may be used to check pain symptoms during exercise.

F. **Stellate ganglion sympathetic blocks** can provide relief of pain due to sympathetic dysfunction. They may be considered for a patient who is refractory to conservative measures. If the first block is moderately effective, a series of 2 or 4 more blocks may be considered to augment other treatment. Stellate ganglion blocks should be performed by an anesthesiologist, physiatrist, orthopedic surgeon, or any other **experienced** physician. Seldom is surgical sympathectomy recommended.

G. **Psychological** problems, such as situational depression, emotional lability, low pain tolerance, and operant behavior, may characterize patients with this syndrome. Care should be taken to assist them through their disabling condition. A clinical psychologist or psychiatrist, however, may be needed to consult on the patient's case.

H. **Home program** involves the active assistance of another person. Paraffin baths, elastic wraps, hand elevation, exercises, and medication usually require help. An occupational therapist can set up and monitor a home program.

Complications. Adhesive capsulitis (so-called frozen shoulder), contractured hand, skin breakdown, chronic pain, lack of limb function, and operant pain behavior can render the patient severely disabled. Aggressive, early intervention is critical in minimizing loss and maximizing recovery.

Adhesive Capsulitis

Adhesive capsulitis is also referred to as frozen shoulder, periarthritis, pericapsulitis, and obliterative bursitis. Its onset is usually insidious. Shoulder pain and restricted joint range of motion characterize the condition, which occurs mainly in people between 50 and 70 years old.

The glenohumeral joint capsule is contractured and adherent to the head of the humerus. Synovial fluid is reduced. The cartilage is normal. Late in the course, osteoporosis of the humeral head may be appreciated on plain radiographs.

Adhesive capsulitis is usually idiopathic. It has been documented with trauma, infection (tuberculosis and isoniazid treatment), thyrotoxicosis, diabetes mellitus, and postmyocardial infarction. It can be a feature of shoulder-hand syndrome.

Evaluation

Pain. The patient may complain of pain in the superior and posterior aspect of the shoulder. Later on, discomfort may be perceived in the neck and shoulder muscles, presumably due to muscle strain. Sleeping on the involved shoulder and moving the shoulder joint aggravate the pain. Although symptoms may abate spontaneously, rest of the shoulder brings prompt pain relief.

Joint Tenderness and Limitation. On palpation, the bicipital groove and acromioclavicular joints may be tender. Range of motion may be particularly lacking toward shoulder abduction, internal rotation, and external rotation. Flexion tends to be less involved.

Arthrography may be necessary to make the diagnosis. Rotator cuff tear, hemarthrosis, infection, aseptic necrosis of the head of the humerus, and anterior capsular rupture often need ruling out.

Management

Depending on the individual case, an intense 6- to 8-week program may be indicated, with sessions as often as 3–5 times per week. An occupational therapist can assist the patient in learning an effective home program and can monitor progress closely.

Pain. During the first 3–5 days of initiating a program, the patient may take an aspirin or a nonsteroidal anti-inflammatory drug (e.g., phenylbutazone). Some physicians prefer prednisone at a dose of 20 mg daily over 5–7 days. A corticosteroid may also be injected into the adherent capsule. Secondarily, pain relief occurs. Analgesics alone do not appear sufficient to control pain. During therapeutic exercise, transcutaneous electrical nerve stimulation may be effective in pain control.

Heat. Although superficial heat may be helpful, there is a clear role for deep heat. Ultrasound is the preferred diathermy. Stretch of the glenohumeral joint should occur during or immediately after treatment.

Motion and Strength. Muscles of the shoulder require conditioning if disuse atrophy is to be minimized. Initially, isometric exercises may restore some strength to the shoulder girdle muscles and relieve the strain of the accessory muscles of the shoulder.

Using passive stretch techniques and a weighted pulley traction, the patient may begin with improving shoulder flexion. External and internal rotation may follow with abduction.

Home Program. The patient should be asked to perform exercises at home three times a day minimally. An occupational therapist may teach the patient the following: "walking" the fingers up the wall; grabbing a pole, cane, or wand with both hands and going through wide motions; glenohumeral pendular, gravity-assisted exercises (Codman); and other related exercises.

Although there may be partial or total remission within 1–3 years, the goal of management is maximal restoration of shoulder function.

Degenerative Tendinitis

This has been referred to as subacromial bursitis, supraspinatus tendinitis, subdeltoid bursitis, and others. The degenerative process involves the rotator cuff (musculotendinous cuff) and the bicipital apparatus. The pain and ache usually develop slowly. The patient grasps the lateral-posterior shoulder to relieve the gnawing pain, especially after attempting shoulder abduction and rotation. Limitation of shoulder range of motion and mild shoulder girdle atrophy may be appreciated. Tenderness is localized to the area of the cuff, not the acromium or bicipital tendon.

An occupational therapist should teach the patient to avoid shoulder abuse or excessive strain **and** to strengthen the shoulder muscles through a home program. The patient should learn proper body mechanics in pushing, pulling, lifting, and elevating objects. Abduction, flexion, rotation (external and internal), and adduction isometric exercises should be taught.

A nonsteroidal anti-inflammatory drug (e.g., phenylbutazone) or a corticosteroid (e.g., predisone, cortisone, triamcinolone) may be prescribed for a 14-day period. An injection of a short-acting anesthetic (lidocaine or procaine 1–2%) 5–10 ml **into the subacromial bursa** may be performed from a posterior approach. The ease of shoulder ranging may improve dramatically. A dose of corticosteroid may be mixed with the anesthetic agent. Transcutaneous electrical nerve stimulation may also be tried.

Rotator Cuff Tear

Overhead movements and relatively minor trauma may rupture the anterior portion of the rotator cuff, particularly in men between 40 and 50 years of age. Typically, pain appears, diminishes, and returns. An incomplete tear may be difficult to diagnose. A complete tear virtually precludes horizontal abduction of the shoulder against manual resistance. Definitive diagnosis may be aided by arthrography, which usually reveals a connection between the glenohumeral capsule and bursa.

In older patients, an incomplete tear may be managed by a splint over 3–4 weeks and abduction isometric exercises. To reduce pain, some physicians recommend mild oral analgesics and an injection of a short-acting anesthetic. In younger patients, a spica case (abducted, externally rotated, forward flexed) may be prescribed by an orthopedic surgeon.

Electrodiagnosis. When involvement of the brachial plexus is suspected by history and clinical examination, electromyography and nerve conduction screens should be considered for precise localization and extent of damage. Prognosis may be greatly aided by electrodiagnostic evidence of denervation or reinnervation.

REFERENCES

Bateman JE, Fornasier VL: The Shoulder and Neck. Philadelphia, Saunders, 1978.
Davis SW et al: Shoulder hand syndrome in a hemiplegic population, a five year retrospective study. Arch Phys Med Rehabil 58:353, 1977.

Leffert RD: Brachial-plexus injuries. New Engl J Med *291*:1059, 1974.
Rizk TE, et al: Adhesive capsulitis (frozen shoulder), a new approach to its management. Arch Phys Med Rehabil *64*:29, 1983.
Subbarao J, Stillwell GK: Reflex sympathetic dystrophy syndrome of the upper extremity. Arch Phys Med Rehabil *62*:549, 1981.
Steinbrocher O: The shoulder-hand syndrome, present perspective. Arch Phys Med Rehabil *49*:388, 1968.

NECK, ELBOW, HAND, AND MYOFASCIAL PAIN

Cervical Radiculopathy

Degenerative disease of the cervical vertebrae and discs develops with age and may produce chronic pain from compression of the cervical nerve root(s). Impingement is more likely to occur when the **neck is extended** or the **head is rotated and flexed laterally** toward the symptomatic side.

The more common sites are C5–6 and C6–7. If the C6 nerve root is pressured, pain and paresthesias may be perceived from the shoulder into the hand, particularly the first two digits. C6-innervated muscle groups may be weaker on careful manual muscle testing. The biceps deep tendon reflex may be less brisk than the contralateral side.

If the C7 nerve root is impinged, symptoms may be felt in the second and third digits. The triceps reflex jerk may be weaker than the other side. In either root compression, passive manipulation of the head and neck toward extension and rotation **toward** the symptomatic side can produce shoulder pain.

Plain radiographs of the cervical spine may reveal signs of degenerative disease but, by themselves, do not substantiate the diagnosis of cervical radiculopathy. CT scan or myelogram may be helpful in selective cases.

Electrodiagnosis is a very useful method of evaluation and should be performed to rule out cervical radiculopathy and other possible dysfunctions of the primary motor unit. The test should be performed 10–14 days after symptoms have begun in order to minimize false-negative results.

Management

Neck and shoulder exercises, proper "body mechanics," and a soft cervical collar may be prescribed to keep muscles in condition, preserve joint range of motion, and remind the patient to avoid sudden movements that exacerbate pain.

Massage and **heat**, superficial or deep, may be applied to paraspinal, neck, and shoulder muscles to alleviate secondary spasm and pain.

The **cervical collar** may be prescribed for 7–14 days during the initial treatment period. The collar should be fitted in **flexion** in a **slightly anterior** direction. Provided the symptoms have subsided, the patient may then begin range-of-motion exercises, initially under supervision. Protracted use of the collar is usually not warranted. It is important to move the patient into a muscle strengthening exercise program and greater active or passive mobility of the head and neck.

Cervical traction may produce significant relief in patients but should not be casually recommended. A **gradual upward and forward pull** tends to distract the posterior elements of the cervical spine and flatten out the lordotic curve. The continual separation of bony elements thereby reduces the mechanical impingement on the cervical nerve root(s). Rhythmic, intermittent traction appears to be more effective than sustained traction. A special device is required and is usually not prescribed for a home traction setup.

Cervical traction is not entirely benign. **Contraindications** include an **unstable vertebral spine** due to trauma; tumor; infection; birth defects; abnormal soft tissue; or rheumatoid arthritis. Severe atherosclerosis of the vertebral or carotid arteries poses special hazards as well. Excessive or sudden jolts to the neck should be avoided. Traction may aggravate or be unnecessary in patients with a fresh neck injury. Even in the patient with the presumably stable cervical spine and chronic radiculopathy, caution should be used. A physical or occupational therapist should methodically teach and assist the patient in a home program. Clinic-based cervical traction requires standby supervision.

Formulas for progressive increments in traction vary from author to author. Starting weight is usually 2.5 kg or 5 lb. Increments daily or every other day average between 1 and 1.5 kg or 2 and 3 lb but range from 0.5–2.5 kg or 1–5 lb. Most patients respond to a total of 9–13 kg, or 20–30 lb. Some patients require up to 16–22 kg, or 35–50 lb. Each session averages between 20 and 30 minutes and occurs daily to three times a week for a 14- to 21-day period. Discontinuation should be gradual.

The patient should assume a reclined position, with steady, firm pull by a halter. The patient's head should be in a slight anterior flexion. The patient should be as relaxed as possible. Cervical traction may be rigged in a doorway at home and consist of a spreader bar, pulley, rope, brackets, and head halter.

Prevention

To minimize the risk of exacerbation or recurrence, the patient should be advised to avoid sudden or prolonged extreme positioning of the neck, particularly in hyperextension. Severe lateral flexion or rotation may also aggravate symptoms. Principles of proper head and neck positioning should be discussed in terms of common daily activities, such as driving the car, sitting at a desk, sleeping, and self-care (dressing, undressing, grooming, hygiene, and bathing). Cleaning, painting, shelving, or constructing areas at home or work that require reaching, stooping, or bending should be mentioned. The appropriate chair, ladder, table, sink, or shelf may enable the patient to use proper body mechanics. Proper posture, however, is not activity-specific but should be assumed at all times. Rounded, hunched-over shoulders are unacceptable. A physical or occupational therapist should teach the patient these guidelines.

Myofascial Pain ("Fibrositis")

The trigger points of myofascial pain are discrete areas of muscle hyperirritability and do not represent an inflammatory process, as the term "fibrositis" denotes. The dull ache, tension, pressure, or pain occurs in the musculature of the back, shoulder, and hip. The origin and insertion of the trapezius muscle (upper portion) at the skull base and scapulae are common sites for palpable, tender trigger points, as are the paraspinal muscles of the cervical spine and back. Interestingly, the patient is usually unaware of the marked tenderness of these points until they are found on discrete palpation.

Management

The patient should be made aware of the contribution made by mental and physical stress, sedentary activities, poor body posture, lack of general exercises, and chronic fatigue. Leg length discrepancy or a Morton foot with a long second metatarsal may aggravate the myofascial ailment. Specific treatment may be indicated for each of these predisposing factors. For example, general conditioning exercises, a firm mattress, a supportive chair at work, and relaxation exercises may be prescribed.

Simple **analgesics** may be taken. **Steroids**, however, should not be taken systematically or injected locally. Muscle relaxants are usually not prescribed.

Fluori-methane spray may effectively distract the patient as vigorous **stretch** of the symptomatic muscle is carried out. The vapocoolant should be sprayed slowly in a stream of parallel "lines." Deep muscle may require anesthetic injection. Peripherally involved muscles with "referred pain" may be treated next. Full range of motion or stretch is important to complete. The cooled skin may be rewarmed with moist superficial heat.

Massage, compressive or kneading, with superficial and deep heat may be tried. Short-wave diathermy may help reduce generalized muscle spasm and facilitate stretch exercises of the involved muscles.

Local injection of **lidocaine** 0.5%–1% **without steroids** may "break up" the reflex irritability of muscle at the trigger points and may be performed at several visits. However effective, injections alone are insufficient without immediate follow-up of coolant spray and muscle stretch.

Epicondylitis

The tennis elbow and golfer's elbow represent overuse syndromes involving the wrist extensor and flexor mechanisms, respectively. They occur with repeated movement at the wrist over a sustained period of time. Tennis, golfing, hammering, hand shaking, and chopping are a few typical activities that can cause epicondylitis.

Rest from the specific activity and time may effectively alleviate symptoms in mild cases. For more intense symptoms, a wrist orthosis and nonsteroidal anti-inflammatory drugs may be prescribed for 2 weeks. An injection of corticosteroid can be administered over the tender and localized area at the elbow. When the medial aspect of the elbow is being injected, the physician should avoid the ulnar nerve. Isometric exercises may strengthen muscles and avoid deconditioning during treatment. It is rare for a patient to require surgery.

de Quervain's Disease

Degenerative disease of the first metacarpophalangeal joint or carpometacarpal joint may cause thumb pain as a result of a stenosing tenosynovitis of the long thumb adductor and short extensor tendons, particularly in the elderly. Carpal tunnel syndrome, degenerative disease of the interphalangeal joint, and rheumatoid arthritis involving other joints may present similarly.

On physical examination, there is tenderness and swelling along the lateral aspect of the radial styloid. When the patient grasps his or her thumb with fingers of the same hand, pain is elicited when the wrist is passively manipulated toward the ulnar direction.

Management

The patient should avoid mechanical stress to the thumb and, if necessary, take aspirin for its analgesic and anti-inflammatory effect. A local injection of a corticosteroid may be considered. A light-weight plastic thumb splint may stabilize the thumb yet allow for interphalangeal flexion of the thumb. An orthotist or occupational therapist may be consulted to fabricate the thumb orthosis.

Carpal Tunnel Syndrome

Compression of the median nerve occurs as it travels under the flexor retinaculum or transverse carpal ligament at the wrist. The clinical outcome is the carpal tunnel syndrome, a prototype of peripheral nerve entrapment disorders.

Its diagnosis consists of symptoms, signs, nerve conduction slowing, and response to splinting. Symptoms include tingling and numbness involving the hand, particularly the first three digits, and occasionally even the arm and shoulder. The latter may falsely suggest a cervical radiculopathy. Symptoms at night are very characteristic.

On physical examination, the patient may have objective loss of pin prick, weakness of median-innervated muscles of the hand, and atrophy of the thenar eminence. Paradoxical hyperflexion at the wrist (Phalen's sign) or percussion at the transverse carpal ligament (Tinel's sign) may produce pain or discomfort.

Electrodiagnosis may reveal delayed distal latencies in the median sensory and motor fibers. Nerve conduction velocity of the forearm segment between elbow and wrist should be normal. A needle electromyogram of the thenar eminence may reveal secondary signs of neurogenic atrophy. A screen of the contralateral wrist may be indicated, since carpal tunnel syndrome is often bilateral in presentation. It should be noted that more proximal entrapment of the median nerve can occur and give the appearance of a carpal tunnel syndrome (anterior interosseous or pronator teres syndrome).

Management

Prompt relief is often obtained with a **cock-up splint** made of plastic or leather. A customized splint may need to be fabricated by an orthotist if commercially available, ready-to-wear ones do not fit properly. **Surgical intervention** is indicated if signs of atrophy have appeared in the muscles or conservative management has failed, or both. The transverse carpal ligament requires complete surgical separation for optimal decompression of the median nerve.

REFERENCES

Cailliet R: Hand Pain and Impairment. Philadelphia, Davis, 1975.
Hunter JM, Schneider LH, Mackin EJ, Bell JA: Rehabilitation of the Hand. St Louis, Mosby, 1978.
Kivi P: Etiology and conservative treatment of humeral epicondylitis. Scand J Rehabil Med 15:37, 1982.

KNEE PAIN

The goals of treatment are **reduced pain, greater strength, joint protection,** and **maximum function. Muscle** rehabilitation should be the foundation of any effort to improve joint stability and function. Painful stimuli may cause reflex inhibition of muscle function. As a result, up to a 30% per week loss in strength may occur in the quadriceps muscle following knee injury and the onset of pain. Protective weight bearing can lead to diffuse weakness of the proximal and distal lower extremities.

Quadriceps weakness results in more mechanical stress about the joint during walking and other weight-bearing activities. The knee depends upon static (ligaments, capsule) and dynamic (musculature) support to compensate for the lack of inherent bony stability.

Poor function of the vastus medialis allows lateral displacement of the patella during flexion and extension of the knee. As a consequence, patellofemoral problems may appear. The loss of dynamic stability is more significant when there is pre-existing ligamentous or capsular laxity due to previous injury or DJD. Nevertheless, muscle strengthening exercises are extremely important to emphasize and carry out.

Muscle Strengthening

Any form of resistance exercise can strengthen the knee, provided there is proper prescription, adequate supervision, and sufficient patient motivation. The key is to **strengthen the muscle without injuring the knee joint.**

Specific programs may incorporate isometric, isotonic, or isokinetic exercises. Repetitive knee flexion and extension movements against resistance may frequently exacerbate symptoms due to chondromalacia or arthritis. In the initial stages, these exercises should be avoided and, in general, seldom prescribed for the knee with chronic pain.

Daily, brief periods of **isometric** contractions are the most effective means of rapid improvement in muscle strength without sacrifice of the joint itself. When **disuse atrophy** without joint pathology is present, however, dynamic resistance exercises are more effective than isometrics. One approach suggests that isometrics be initiated first. When pain-free movement against resistance is possible, isotonic or isokinetic exercises may begin.

Isometric Quadriceps Sets

This exercise is most effective when performed once or twice daily. Do not instruct patients to "tighten the thigh muscle 10 times each hour." It is not physiologic, realistic, or efficacious. The knee should be maximally extended for 8 seconds, alternating 2 seconds of rest over a 3- to 5-minute session b.i.d. Voluntary effort may be improved by the patient if he or she does the following:

1. Uses a watch or metronome.
2. Palpates the vastus medialis during contraction.
3. Looks in a mirror for visual feedback.
4. Elevates the heel above the floor to minimize cheating.

5. Concentrates on increasing muscle tension with each second count.

6. Avoids breath holding; or, counts out loud.

The thigh should feel tight or ache slightly following adequate exercise.

Straight Leg Raising

Straight leg raising augments quadriceps sets and may hasten the transition to isotonic strengthening exercises. The knee is locked in extension. The leg is raised slowly up and down through an arc of about 30 degrees. Weights are usually fixed to the lower leg or foot. Three to five sets of 10–20 repetitions per set are performed with 1-minute rest periods between each set. The weight may be increased as tolerated weekly until a maximum of 30 lb is reached. Beyond 30 lb, the additional stress on the hip flexors and low back can become deleterious. At that point, the patient may graduate to isotonic exercises.

Isotonic Knee Extension

This exercise is performed against progressive resistance on a knee extension table. Alternatively, weights may be attached to the foot or ankle. A successful weight lifting protocol utilizes an initial warm-up period. Next, the patient uses the maximum weight to carry out 10 repetitions. As the weight is increased, the number of repetitions is progressively decreased until 3–5 sets with maximum muscle fatigue is attained.

For example, the patient may warm up with 15 repetitions and 20 lb; then, 10 repetitions, 30 lb; then, 7 repetitions, 40 lb; then, 5 repetitions, 50 lb. The patient takes 1-minute rests between sets and exercises daily. The weights are increased weekly. A written record should be kept.

If **patellofemoral pain** is present, this exercise should be limited to the last 15–30 degrees of extension, or short arc extensions. The reduction in flexion can decrease patellofemoral compression without compromising improvement of vastus medialis strength. A small stool or bench can be placed under the exercised extremity in order to limit knee flexion.

This method of increasing resistance with each set (DeLorme) is recommended over the technique of decreasing resistance (Oxford). If heavy weights are lifted without adequate warm-up, soft tissue or joint injury is more likely to happen. The former method tends to reach maximum fatigue and thereby improves strength more efficiently.

Isokinetic Method

Special equipment (Cybex or Orthotron) is utilized to control the rate of joint movement. The amount of resistance (torque) is dependent on the patient's effort and is directly measurable on the machine. The isokinetic machine can accommodate a specific area in the range of motion where pain is elicited by maximal effort. The direct graphic feedback may be positively reinforcing. Muscle ache tends to be less because only concentric (shortening) contractions against resistance are permitted.

In peripatellar pain syndrome, the full knee extension range of motion may be tolerated by the isokinetic method. The patient is able to lessen effort through the few degrees of patellar pain and gives full effort through the remainder of pain-free range of motion. This may more effectively develop quadriceps strength than the isotonic method. In the latter, the maximum amount of resistance is limited by that which can be tolerated through the arc of pain.

The isokinetic technique utilizes an expensive machine and requires proper supervision by a specially trained physical therapist.

A muscle strengthening program should maximize the function of the quadriceps muscles, as well as that of the hamstrings and gastrocnemius-soleus muscles. Other, more proximal or distal muscle groups may need conditioning. If the chronic pain bothers only one knee, the therapeutic goal should be symmetric strength in the lower extremities.

Activity Modifications

Most cases of chronic knee pain respond to **rest** or **reduced physical activity.** Complete rest for a few days may prepare the patient for a full exercise program. **Immobilization** is sometimes necessary for a clearly defined and limited period of time. Isometric exercises b.i.d.–q.i.d. should be recommended to minimize atrophy and further muscle weakness. An acute flare of rheumatoid arthritis or Osgood-Schlatter disease may respond to immobilization and not rest alone.

When pain is clearly related to a specific activity, a change in that activity is desirable. For example, runners with chronic knee pain should decrease daily mileage, avoid pavements, run on level ground, exercise every other day, or discontinue running completely for brief periods of several days or more.

In patients with rheumatoid arthritis or DJD, stair climbing, squatting, heavy lifting, and long distance walking should be avoided when symptoms are more intense.

Therapeutic Cold and Heat

Cold

Ice towel, ice bath, or ice massage may be applied at home and followed by range of motion and other appropriate exercises. Ice frozen in styrofoam cups may be applied to the area of tenderness (e.g., patellar tendinitis) with light brushing strokes back and forth for about 5–10 minutes (depending on the size of the area) until numbness is perceived. If pain persists, the ice massage may be repeated. The therapy may be recommended b.i.d.–q.i.d.

Superficial Heat

Moist warm towels may be applied over the knee and changed every 5–10 minutes during a 30- to 60-minute treatment session at home. A brief 10- to 15-minute session may be sufficient to relieve pain and anxiety prior to muscle strengthening exercises in a patient with arthritis or chronic patellar pain syndrome. Avoid scalding burns. Avoid vigorous heat in an acute arthritic joint. Warm baths may relax muscles in spasm and, in addition, provide buoyancy that may encourage greater joint movement.

Orthotics and Walking Aids

Devices for external support of the knee may be necessary to alleviate pain, provide stability, and limit deformity during standing, walking, and other weight-bearing activity.

Knee-ankle-foot orthoses (so-called long leg braces) may be prescribed for a patient with severe DJD (see the section on bracing the lower extremity).

Knee cages extend from just above to just below the knee to prevent genu recurvatum. They may be effective for standing transfers and short distance walking. They tend to slip with more demanding activity.

Knee braces are characterized by hinged metal medial-lateral stays and elastic wraps, which provide medial-lateral stability and protect the knee following collateral ligament injury. The Lenox-Hill is an example of a knee brace. Some physicians contend that the brace "reminds" the patient to avoid excessive knee stress rather than provides external substitution of weakened knee structures. The knee cage should never be considered an alternative to adequate muscle strengthening.

A **patellar brace** is usually a rubberized knee sleeve and an anterior well to accommodate the patella. A lateral wedge may be preferred to prevent lateral displacement of the patella. Symptomatic relief may occur in patients with patellar instability or chondromalacia, particularly during exercise.

A **patellar strap** may be as effective as a patellar brace. A leather or elastic strap with Velcro stays may be wrapped around the knee at the inferior aspect of the patella. This alteration of the patellofemoral mechanism may reduce the symptoms of chondromalacia during exercise.

Knee splints may be recommended to immobilize the knee. Plaster, fiberglass, plastic, or metal splints can be custom-molded by an orthotist or cast technician. Some splints may be purchased as "shelf-items." These splints may be prescribed for patients with severe knee arthritis as night-resting splints.

Arch support for the foot may prevent excessive subtalar joint pronation in patients with chronic knee pain and obvious rotatory malalignment of the lower extremity. Scholl's 611 or Roberts rear foot controls may be tried before going to custom-molded plastic supports.

Chronic Anterior Knee Pain

Peripatellar pain is the most frequent presenting complaint of knee pain in primary care. Those cases involving the extensor mechanism include chondromalacia patellae, patellar instability, patellar compression, patellar tendinitis, Osgood-Schlatter disease, and medial retinaculitis. Other causes include torn medial meniscus, infrapatellar fat pad lesion, infrapatellar tendon bursitis, suprapatellar plica, osteochondral fractures, osteochondritis dissecans, iliotibial band friction syndrome, and pes anserinus bursitis.

Chondromalacia

In chondromalacia, the undersurface articular cartilage of the patella softens, and fissures are most often due to trauma or abnormal patellofemoral mechanics. Symptoms occur frequently in adolescents and young adults but may be seen in older age groups. Peripatellar ache increases in going down steps or hills, prolonged sitting with knee flexion, or following exercise.

There may be catching, grating, transient "locking," swelling, stiffness, instability, or giving way. Patellar facet tenderness, crepitation, and a positive patellar inhibition sign may be present. Femoral anteversion, squinting patella, tibial varum, external tibial torsion, increased compensatory subtalar joint pronation with pes planus, and other malalignments may be found. The quadriceps angle (Q angle) is often increased (greater than 10 degrees in males and 15 degrees in females) and is measured at the intersection of these lines from the center of the patella to the anterior superior iliac spine and the tibial tubercle. Quadriceps weakness or atrophy of the vastus medialis may be present. Tangential radiographs of the knee may indicate an increased sulcus angle, decreased lateral femoral condyle, or abnormal patella.

Treatment is directed at reduction of symptoms, restoration of quadriceps strength, and graduated return to activity on a maintenance program. In less than 10% of cases, surgery is necessary to revise the patellofemoral mechanics.

Symptomatic pain relief may be achieved by restricting activities and by giving salicylates. Complete bed rest and avoidance of specific exacerbating activities may be necessary. Complete immobilization, however, is rarely indicated. Stair climbing, squatting, and prolonged sitting with flexed knees may provide mild symptomatic relief. Substitute physical activities and limited rest may be recommended for 2–6 weeks, depending on the individual case. Aspirin therapy over 2–6 weeks usually reduces the pain.

Vastus medialis strength should be improved without aggravation of patellar pain. Preceded by a period of rest and aspirin, daily quadriceps sets and straight leg raising exercises may begin the exercise program. A physical therapist or athletic trainer may be consulted to teach and supervise this program, which subsequently involves short arc extensions, isotonic hamstring exercises, and strengthening of other muscle groups of the hip, knee, and ankle.

Most patients experience significant relief of discomfort within 2–6 weeks. In severe cases, symptoms may persist for several months. Restriction and gradual return to specific activities depend on the individual patient. As a rule, vigorous young athletes may return to unrestricted activity when they can perform leg extensions with about one third of their body weight with each leg. If symptoms involve only one knee, their weaker quadriceps should be 10% or less in strength than the normal, stronger knee.

Orthotic foot controls may be useful in patients with significant rotatory malalignment. Proper fitting shoes are critical. For example, the best street shoes are usually made of firm leather uppers, heels, and soles. Neoprene soles are often substituted. A patellar brace or strap may be indicated for running or jumping.

After the patient returns to full activity, a maintenance program of short arc extension 3 times a week or isometric quadriceps sets daily should be encouraged. Activities that provoke symptoms should be restricted or avoided. Aspirin should be taken as necessary. After a 6-month conservative management, surgery may be considered.

Other Patellar Pain

Other causes of chronic patellar pain are managed by similar principles of appropriate rest, aspirin, specific exercises, orthotics, graduated activity, and maintenance for prevention. The discussion of each entity, however, is beyond the scope of this manual. Note that there are exceptions, such as the aggravation of pain caused by quadriceps exercises in acute patellar tendinitis or Osgood-Schlatter disease. A physiatrist or orthopedist may be consulted to assist in the evaluation and management.

Degenerative Joint Disease

This degenerative disease is the most common knee disability with advancing age. Repetitive trauma aggravates joint instability and deformity. Deep aches may occur after arduous activity or prolonged rest. Effusion, creptitation, stiffness, tenderness, angular deformity, and limited joint range of motion often characterize the affected knee. Loss of joint space, bony sclerosis, subchondral cysts, and marginal osteophytes may be seen on plain radiographs.

Patients should learn to **minimize joint stress** by modifying activities, losing weight, changing the home environment, wearing orthoses, or using walking aids. Long walks, stair climbing, rough ground, heavy lifting, and low chairs should be avoided. Proper arm chair, raised toilet seat, tub bench, and grab bars in the bathroom may greatly help the patient.

Isometric exercises of the quadriceps and other muscle groups of the hips, knees, and ankles should be considered for proper teaching, supervision, and monitoring by a physical therapist. With severe genu varus or valgus, knee-ankle-foot orthoses may be recommended by a physiatrist or orthopedist.

Pain relief may be attained by aspirin or other nonsteroidal anti-inflammatory drugs (e.g., indomethacin, naproxen). The prescribing physician should be thoroughly familiar with the adverse side effects of these drugs and monitor the patient's response to them carefully. Superficial heat and hydrotherapy may be effective. Symptoms refractory to conservative measures may warrant surgical osteotomy or joint replacement.

Rheumatoid Arthritis

Acute flare-ups require rest and immobilization, which should be less than 2–4 weeks to minimze loss of joint motion and further muscle atrophy. Positioning of the affected limb is important. For example, pillows should not be propped under the knee, since this promotes flexion contracture at the knee, hip, and ankle. Orthoses should be removable to allow for gentle passive range of motion on a daily basis.

In the acute phase, cold may be applied over the knee to reduce pain and inflammation. In more chronic stages, superficial or deep heat may be applied prior to range of motion and strengthening exercises.

Because rheumatoid arthritis of the knee invariably leads to weakness of the extensor mechanism, patients should be advised to perform isometric exercises daily. Short arc extensions without pain may be done to strengthen the vastus medialis. Isotonic exercises with heavy resistance should be avoided.

Special orthoses may be considered for patients with marked instability and deformity in the knee(s). A knee-ankle-foot orthosis with a knee hinge can decrease the stress of weight bearing and maintain joint alignment. In less severe cases, a knee cage may prevent excessive backknee and provide some medial-lateral stability for short distance walking.

Walking aids can provide considerable relief of troubled weight-bearing joints. When the upper extremities are severely afflicted with arthritis, a crutch or walker with forearm support may be prescribed.

Neuromuscular disorders and knee management are discussed elsewhere in this manual.

FOOT AND ANKLE PAIN

The successful management of chronic foot pain requires an understanding of the functional anatomy and biomechanics, particularly in walking, alignment of the lower extremities, and position of the subtalar joint.

Shoes

The shoe may be regarded as an orthosis that protects and supports the foot. Deformities, in addition, may be accommodated or corrected. Improper selection or inadequate fit can aggravate chronic foot symptoms, as well as create new problems.

A well-designed shoe should provide arch support, even weight distribution at the ball of the foot, and adequate room for the ball of the foot and the toes. The shoe should fit firmly around the ankle and midfoot to minimize excessive motion and provide support. The first metatarsal head should be located at the break in the shoe.

Length, width, height, and construction (upper, heel, and sole) should be considered. An ideal prototype is a leather oxford style with leather upper, firm heel counter, and wide toe box. The leather sole should have a steel shank from midheel to the ball of the foot. Such a prototype accommodates modifications and inserts without sacrificing support.

Styles of shoes and common chronic complaints. A good quality leather oxford may significantly relieve symptoms of constantly tired, aching feet often found in people who stand long hours at work. As the leather soles conform more to the shape of the foot, greater comfort is usually experienced.

For patients with bunions, metatarsalgia, arthritic deformity, toe abnormalities, or pes planus, crepe or rippled-sole shoes may aggravate discomfort or pain. Although they improve traction and absorb shock better, the soft sole provides less stability and increases shear forces during ambulation.

High heels increase weight bearing on the metatarsal heads and toes and aggravate painful symptoms. Negative heels, on the other hand, may increase symptoms by placing abnormal stress on the subtalar joint or Achilles tendon. Patients should consider a flat sole with a heel lift or a standard ¾-in. heel.

Western boots and other pointed shoe styles do not have an adequate toe box. The first metatarsal head rubs against the medial aspect of the shoe in full weight bearing. Thus, chronic symptoms from bunions, toe deformities, splayed forefoot, and other abnormalities are exacerbated. Ideally, the toe box should be high enough to eliminate pressure on the proximal interphalangeal joint when flexion deformities exist. As a rule, the length of the toe box should allow for 1 in. of toe clearance.

Shoe Modification

A **metatarsal bar** relieves weight-bearing stress on the metatarsal heads during standing and walking. A ⅛-in. leather bar is placed behind the metatarsal heads. The shoe pivots over the bar and effectively decreases the amount of dorsiflexion required at the metatarso-phalangeal joint. A metatarsal bar may be helpful in pes cavus, hallux rigidus, and metatarsalgia. It is a short-term solution to a problem. Patients should be cautioned that they may initially tend to trip over uneven surfaces.

A **rocker bottom** functions much the same as a metatarsal bar. It may compensate well for immobilization of a fused ankle or forefoot. The rocker bottom may be considered as a more permanent solution to pain from problems of the metatarsal heads or metatarsophalangeal joint.

A **Thomas heel** is a medial extension of the heel to increase the weight-bearing surface. In pes planus, the heel increases support of the medial longitudinal arch and decreases pronation. A reverse Thomas heel or lateral heel flare compensates for a fixed heel varus.

A valgus or T-strap may be recommended when excessive heel valgus results from abnormal medial-lateral alignment of the ankle due to spasticity or muscle contracture. The strap is usually incorporated into a prescription for an ankle-foot orthosis (so-called short leg brace).

Inserts

Inserts are prescribed to provide better foot positioning and to relieve pressure. They range from simple to custom-molded appliances.

Heel cups or **heel pads** cushion the heel. Chronic pain from Sever's apophysitis, fat pad loss with aging, and subtalar joint arthritis may be managed this way. A **doughnut pad** with cutout may be placed directly under the point of tenderness in such conditions as a heel spur in plantar fasciitis.

The choice of **arch supports** depends on the amount of support and degree of pronation control that are most appropriate for the patient. Arch cookies and navicular pads may be fashioned out of surgical felt, neoprene, Spenco rubber, cork, or other materials. Scholl's 611, Robert's rear foot controls, and other over-the-counter arch supports can provide adequate support when they fit properly.

Custom arch supports of flexible or rigid material may modify the duration of pronation during gait. Custom leather supports wear out more frequently than more expensive rigid controls. For the control of pronation at the subtalar joint, firm or rigid plastic supports should be considered. Less expensive supports should be tried initially because even customized plastic supports do not always work. Patients who stand long hours over hard surfaces and long distance runners with overuse symptoms secondary to hyper-pronation may benefit from them.

Low dye strapping and other taping methods may help to maintain the arch and limit pronation. These may be tried to determine whether or not orthotic controls are likely to provide symptomatic relief.

Shoe depth must be adequate to accommodate arch supports without the loss of purchase for support around the heel and midfoot. Laced shoe styles should be preferred over slip-ons. A removable inner sole, firm heel counter, straight lasts, and wide toe box characterize shoes that provide excellent arch support in runners.

A special arch support, pads, and plastic inserts may be prescribed for a patient with chronic pain due to metatarsal head pathology. A **Morton's extension** is simply an arch support designed to encompass the first metatarsal head. Soft **metatarsal pads** may be placed posterior to the metatarsal heads. Or, **plastozote,** a moldable polyethylene plastic, may be shaped to the individual foot to limit weight-bearing stress on the metatarsal heads.

Orthoses

A **patellar tendon bearing** orthosis is a special brace with a cuff below the knee that functions to transmit weight bearing of the distal tibia, ankle, and foot proximally onto the patellar tendon area. It may be useful in the management of chronic problems from a fused ankle, arthritis, nonunion, intractable heel pain, heel fractures, Charcot joints, and painful neuropathic ulcerations.

Ankle-foot orthoses are discussed in other sections in this manual.

Therapeutic Exercises

Exercises can play a major role in the management of chronic painful conditions of the foot and ankle. Recurrent ankle sprains and chronic instability may be helped by daily exercises to strengthen the invertors, evertors, dorsiflexors, and plantar flexors of the ankle and foot. Exercises may include repetitive movement against surgical tubing resistance, sustained isometric contractions, walking exercises with feet inverted or everted, and activating the intrinsic muscles of the foot to pick up beach balls, pencils, and other small objects. Similarly, chronic foot strain from pes planus may be helped with strengthening exercises of the intrinsic musculature.

In chronic arthritis and other conditions that limit joint range of motion, daily ranging should be performed. Stretch of the gastrocnemius-soleus and peroneal muscles may be recommended for increased heel valgus, subtalar joint pronation, or fallen arches.

Management of Common Disorders

Chronic Ankle Pain

When a patient acutely re-injures a **chronically unstable ankle,** ice, compression, elevation, and rest for 48–72 hours are recommended. A cast or other protective weight-bearing device should be worn until the patient is pain-free. Concomitantly, a program of muscle strengthening and gradual return to activity should be instituted and may last from a few weeks to several months. The clinical goal is a return to pain-free activity.

Prolonged immobilization predisposes the patient to significant loss in strength, joint range, and proprioception. A splint or tape can be removed daily to permit exercises. Contrast baths may be prescribed with exercises. The patient moves from isometric to isotonic exercises with emphasis on the peroneals, anterior tibial, posterior tibial, and gastrocnemius-soleus muscles.

Weight bearing begins slowly. When walking becomes pain-free, activity may expand. Taping or splinting should be worn to continue ankle protection and minimize the risk of re-injury.

In **arthritis,** a softer heel wedge or heel cup may increase shock absorption at heel strike. With decreased ankle motion, a rocker bottom or rigid shank should be considered. Medial and lateral flares may compensate for valgus or varus deformities, respectively.

A **Charcot joint** due to a neuropathic arthropathy may be managed by a patellar tendon–bearing orthosis. The floppy ankle from **common peroneal palsy** may be painful from chronic joint instability. A plastic ankle-foot orthosis may be prescribed.

Rear Foot Pain

Chronic or recurrent Achilles tendinitis may be initially treated with ice, aspirin, and rest. Stretch of the gastrocnemius-soleus muscles should be faithfully done before and after vigorous exercises. A heel lift may decrease stress on the tendon. For excessive pronation, arch supports should be considered. Exostosis or bursitis may require a change in shoes. The heel counter may be higher or perpendicular; a heel cup may be helpful. Surgical felt may be cut out to relieve areas of pressure. Gradual return to activities should occur with a decrease or elimination of symptoms.

Other causes of heel pain, such as Sever's apophysitis or calcaneal epiphysitis, can be managed in principle in a similar way. Knowledge of the pathology, however, is important.

Midfoot Pain

Plantar fasciitis and **chronic foot strain** are common disorders of chronic pain of the midfoot or arch. Anterior medial heel pain radiates into the arch and varies directly with activity. Its insidious onset is usually associated with prolonged standing, walking, or running. The proximal medial arch and the anterior medial heel (should an osteophyte be present) are usually tender.

Patients with plantar fasciitis respond to rigid plastic inserts. A medial heel wedge or heel cutout, however, may be tried initially. For chronic foot strain, management should include properly fitting shoes, custom-molded arch supports, and, occasionally, medial heel wedges or extensions. Exercises should strengthen muscle, stretch the gastrocnemius-soleus muscles, and emphasize toe grip and supination during walking.

Chronic Forefoot Pain

Gout, rheumatoid arthritis, trauma, infection, DJD, hallux rigidus, hallux valgus (common bunion), and sesamoiditis may cause chronic or recurrent pain in the forefoot. Pressure relief under the first metatarsophalangeal joint may be achieved by a larger toe box, leather sole, metatarsal pad, arch support, steel shank, rocker bottom, or a combination of them.

Metatarsalgia presents with dull aching or cramping occurring with walking, especially at push-off. Recent weight gain, prolonged standing on hard surfaces, and other overuse activities predispose patients to tenderness over the metatarsal heads, particularly the third and fourth. Metatarsalgia is often associated with a broad foot, weak intrinsic muscles, or foot deformities. It may be managed by metatarsal bar or pad proximal to the metatarsal heads acutely. Intrinsic muscle strengthening, arch supports, gastrocnemius-soleus stretch, wide shoes, weight loss, and restricted activity may be indicated. Metatarsalgia should be differentiated.

Morton's neuroma (plantar digital neuroma) may appear with metatarsalgic symptoms. However, cramping appears in the anterior foot with paresthesias extending into the toes. Weight bearing, toe extension, and squeezing the digits together usually provoke symptoms of pain or tenderness.

Hammertoes and **clawtoes** may form painful calluses and may be accommodated by proper shoes and routine callus care.

Consultation may be sought from an orthopedist, physiatrist, orthotist, physical therapist, podiatrist, athletic trainers, and other professionals who have experience and interest in the management of chronic foot and ankle pain.

REFERENCE

Zamosky I, Licht S, Redford JB: Shoes and their modification, Chap 11, pp. 368–431. In Redford JB (ed): Orthotics Etcetera, 2nd ed. Baltimore, Williams & Wilkins, 1980.

V

APPENDICES

V

APPENDICES

1

RESOURCES

The following list of resources represents only a small portion of the numerous organizations, agencies, programs, foundations, and periodicals focused on physically disabled people. Each general or specialized resource usually has a list of printed material, newsletters, videotapes, or films for free, loan, or purchase.

ORGANIZATIONS

American Academy of Physical Medicine and Rehabilitation, 30 North Michigan Avenue, Chicago, Illinois 60602.

American Congress of Rehabilitation Medicine, 30 North Michigan Avenue, Chicago, Illinois 60602.

Disabled American Veterans, National Headquarters, PO Box 1403, Cincinnati, Ohio 45214.

Disabled Resources Center, 330 East Broadway Street, Long Beach, California 90802.

Human Resources Center, Willets Road, Albertson, New York 11507.

National Association of the Physically Handicapped, 2810 Terrace Road SE, Washington, DC 20020.

National Easter Seal Society for Crippled Children and Adults, 2023 West Ogden Avenue, Chicago, Illinois 60612.

National Congress of Organizations of the Physically Handicapped, 6105 North 30th St., Arlington, Virginia 22207.

Office of Special Education and Rehabilitative Services, National Institute of Handicapped Research, Department of Education, Washington, DC 20202.

National Foundation of Dentistry for the Handicapped, 1121 Broadway Street, Suite 5, Boulder, Colorado 80302.

National Rehabilitation Association, 1522 K Street NW, Washington, DC 20005.

National Information Center for the Handicapped, 1201 16th Street SW, Washington, DC 20036.

National Rehabilitation Information Center, 308 Mullen Library, Catholic University of America, Washington DC 20004.

Programs for the Handicapped, Office for Handicapped Individuals, Switzer Building, Room 3517, 330 C Street SW, Washington, DC 20201.

International Society for Rehabilitation of the Disabled, 432 Park Avenue South, New York, New York 10016.

Rehabilitation International, USA, 20 West 40th Street, New York, New York 10018.

Rehabilitation Engineering Society of North America, 4405 East-West Highway, Suite 210, Bethesda, Maryland 20814.

ORGANIZATIONS FOR SPECIFIC PHYSICAL DISABILITIES

Amyotrophic lateral sclerosis: A. L. S. Foundation, 15300 Ventura Boulevard, Suite 315, Sherman Oaks, California 91463.

Amputation
Amputees' Service Association, Suite 1504, 520 North Michigan Avenue, Chicago, Illinois 60611.
National Amputation Foundation, 12–45 150th Street, White Stone, New York 11357.

Arthritis: Arthritis Foundation, 1212 Avenue of the Americas, New York, New York 10036.

Arthrogryposis: Avenues, 5430 East Harbor Heights Drive, Port Orchard, Washington 98366.

Cerebral palsy
United Cerebral Palsy Associations, 66 East 34th Street, New York, New York 10016.
The Spastics Society, 12 Park Crescent, London W1N 4LQ, England.
American Academy for Cerebral Palsy and Developmental Medicine, PO Box 11083, Richmond, Virginia 23230.

Cerebrovascular disease
Cardio-Vascular Disease, American Heart Association, 44 East 23rd Street, New York, New York 10010.
Stroke Clubs of America, 805 12th Street, Galveston, Texas 77550.

Congenital defects: National Foundation/March of Dimes, PO Box 2000, White Plains, New York 10605.

Dwarfism: Little People of America, PO Box 126, Owatonna, Minnesota 55060.

Friedreich's ataxia: Friedreich's Ataxia Group in America, Box 1116, Oakland, California 94611.

Head injury: National Head Injury Foundation, 18A Vernon Street, Framingham, Massachusetts 01701.

Hemophilia: National Hemophilia Foundation, 25 West 39th Street, New York, New York 10018.

Multiple sclerosis
Association to Overcome Multiple Sclerosis (ATOMS), 79 Milk Street, Boston, Massachusetts 02109.
National Multiple Sclerosis Society, 205 East 42nd Street, New York, New York 10010.

Muscular dystrophy: Muscular Dystrophy Associations of America, 810 Seventh Avenue, New York, New York 10019.

Myasthenia gravis: Myasthenia Gravis Foundation, 2 East 103rd Street, New York, New York 10029.

Myelomeningocele and spina bifida

Spina Bifida Association, The Texas Medical Center, 2333 Moursund Street, Houston, Texas 77025.

Spina Bifida Association of America, 104 Festone Avenue, New Castle, Delaware 19720.

Ostomies: United Ostomy Association, 1111 Wilshire Boulevard, Los Angeles, California 90017.

Parkinson's disease

American Parkinson's Disease Association, 116 John Street, New York, New York 10038.

United Parkinson Foundation, 220 South State Street, Chicago, Illinois 60604.

Spinal cord injury

National Paraplegia Foundation, 333 North Michigan Avenue, Chicago, Illinois 60601.

Paralyzed Veterans of America, 7315 Wisconsin Avenue NW, Washington, DC 20014.

PUBLICATIONS AND PERIODICALS

Accent on Living, PO Box 726, Gillum Road and High Drive, Bloomington, Illinois 61701.

DAV (See Disabled American Veterans)

Disabled, USA, President's Committee for Employment of the Handicapped, Washington, DC 20210.

Green Pages, PO Box 1586, Winter Park, Florida 32289.

The Independent, Center for Independent Living, 2539 Telegraph Road, Berkeley, California 94704.

Office of Publications, Institute of Rehabilitation Medicine, New York University Medical Center, 400 East 34th Street, New York, New York 10016.

International Rehabilitation Review, 219 East 44th Street, New York, New York 10017.

Journal of Rehabilitation (See National Rehabilitation Association)

Media Resources Branch, National Medical Audiovisual Center, Annex-Station K, Atlanta, Georgia 30324.

Paraplegia Life (See National Paraplegia Foundation)

Paraplegia News, 5201 North 19th Avenue, Suite 108, Phoenix, Arizona 85015.

Polling, United Cerebral Palsy Associations, 122 East 23rd Street, New York, New York 10010.

Public Affairs Pamphlets, 381 Park Avenue South, New York, New York 10016.

Rehabilitation Gazette, 4502 Maryland Avenue, St. Louis, Missouri 63108.

Rehabilitation Literature (See Easter Seal Society)

Rehabilitation World (See Rehabilitation International)

RPG-REHAB Purchasing Guide, 1983, IMS Press, 426 Pennsylvania Avenue, Fort Washington, Pennsylvania 19034.

Office of Publications, Sister Kenny Institute, 1800 Chicago Avenue, Minneapolis, Minnesota 55407.

Sports 'n Spokes (See Paralyzed Veterans of America)

Superintendent of Documents, United States Government Printing Office, Washington, DC 20402.

Velleman RA: Serving Physically Disabled People, An Information Handbook for All Libraries. New York, RR Bowker, 1979.

2

JOINT RANGE OF MOTION

Reproduced with the permission of the Committee for the Study of Joint Motion. Joint Motion—Method of Measuring and Recording. Chicago, American Academy of Orthopaedic Surgeons, 1965.

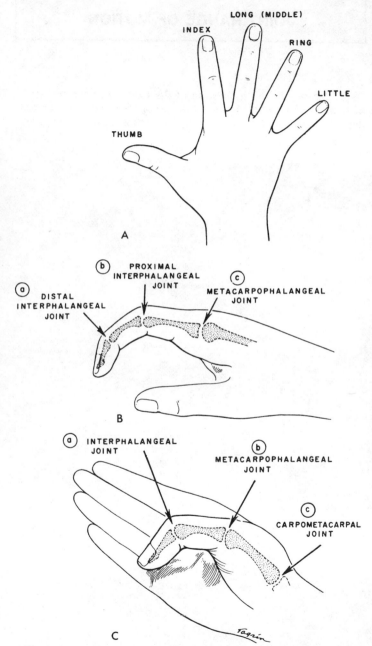

Figure A–1. The hand. *A*, Nomenclature of the fingers. *B*, Joints of the fingers. *C*, Joints of the thumb.

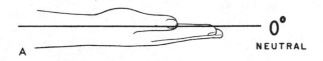

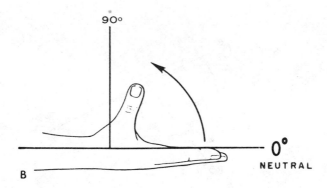

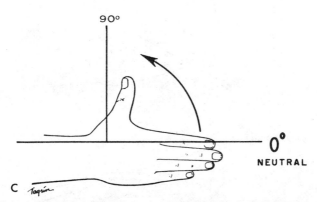

Figure A–2. The thumb (circumduction and abduction). *A,* Zero starting position. *B,* Circumduction at right angle to the plane of the palm. *C,* Extension parallel to the plane of the palm.

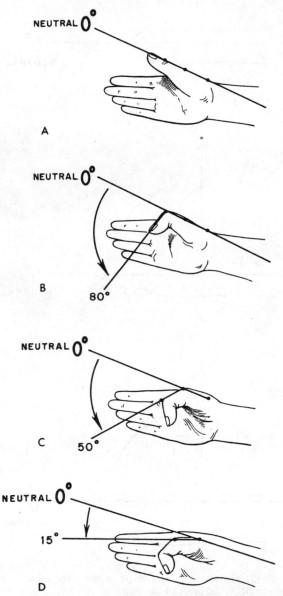

Figure A–3. The thumb (flexion). *A*, Zero starting position. *B*, Interphalangeal joint. *C*, Metacarpophalangeal joint. *D*, Carpometacarpal joint.

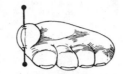

ZERO STARTING POSITION

① ABDUCTION

② ROTATION

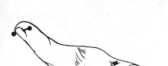

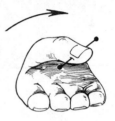

③ and FLEXION

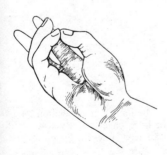

OR

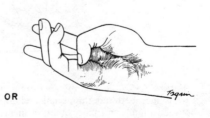

FLEXION TO TIP OF
LITTLE FINGER

FLEXION TO BASE OF
LITTLE FINGER

Figure A–4. The thumb (opposition): composite of three motions.

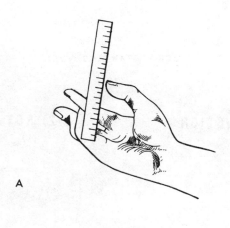

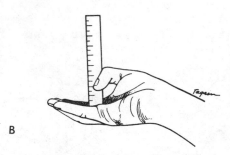

Figure A–5. The thumb: measurement of limitation of opposition. *A,* By distance between thumbnail and top of little finger. *B,* By distance between thumb and base of little finger. (Advice: "Use 5th finger when present.")

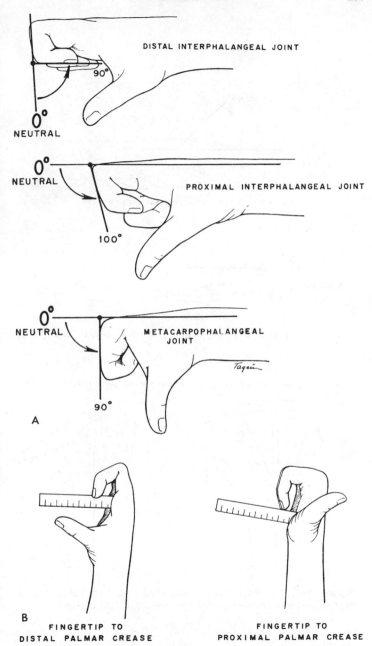

Figure A–6. The fingers (flexion). *A*, Flexion. *B*, Composite motion of flexion.

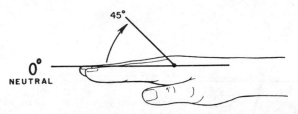

EXTENSION - METACARPOPHALANGEAL JOINT

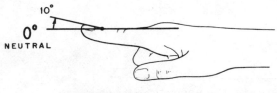

HYPEREXTENSION - DISTAL INTERPHALANGEAL JOINT

A

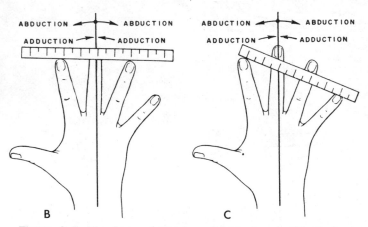

B   C

Figure A–7. The fingers (extension, abduction, and adduction). *A,* Extension and hyperextension. *B,* Finger spread. *C,* Other fingers.

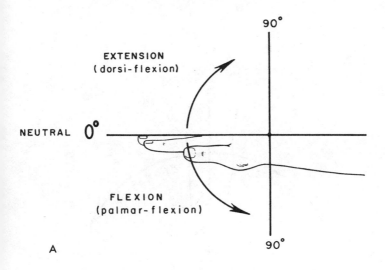

90°

EXTENSION
(dorsi-flexion)

NEUTRAL 0°

FLEXION
(palmar-flexion)

90°

A

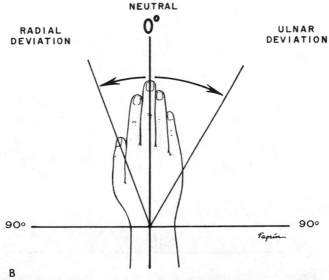

NEUTRAL
0°

RADIAL
DEVIATION

ULNAR
DEVIATION

90°   90°

B

Figure A–8. The wrist. *A*, Flexion and extension. *B*, Radial and ulnar deviation.

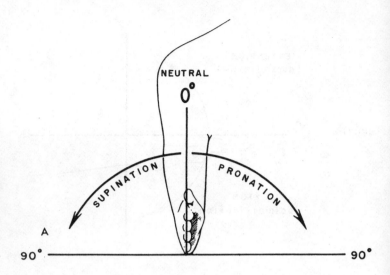

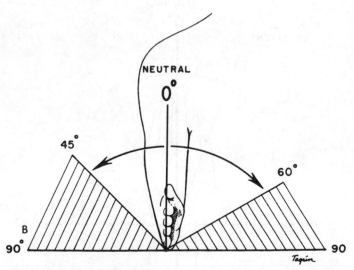

Figure A–9. The forearm (elbow and wrist). *A*, Pronation and supination. *B*, Measurement of limited motion.

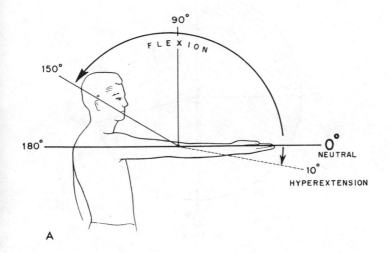

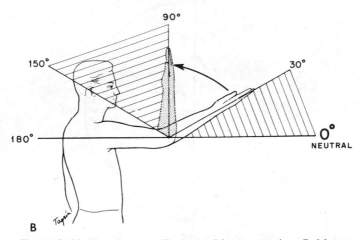

Figure A–10. The elbow. *A,* Flexion and hyperextension. *B,* Measurement of limited motion.

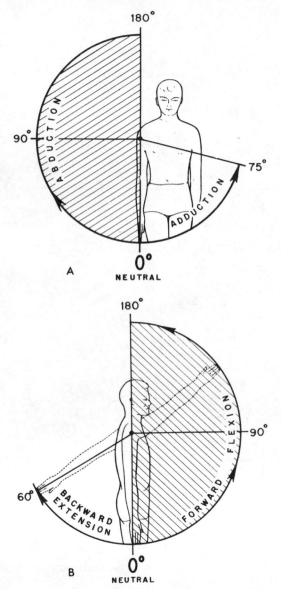

Figure A–11. Motion of the arm at the shoulder. *A*, Abduction and adduction (in vertical plane). *B*, Forward flexion and backward extension (in vertical plane).

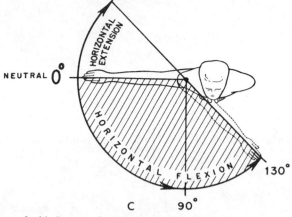

Figure A–11 *Continued. C,* Horizontal flexion (in horizontal plane).

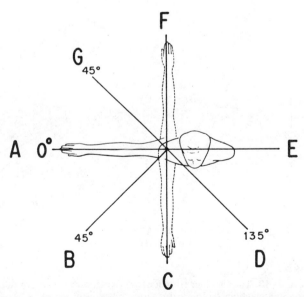

Figure A–12. The shoulder: terminology identifying upward motion of the arm in various horizontal positions. *Positions: A,* Neutral abduction; *B,* abduction in 45° of horizontal flexion; *C,* forward flexion; *D,* adduction in 135° of horizontal flexion; *E,* neutral adduction; *F,* backward extension; *G,* abduction in 45° of horizontal extension.

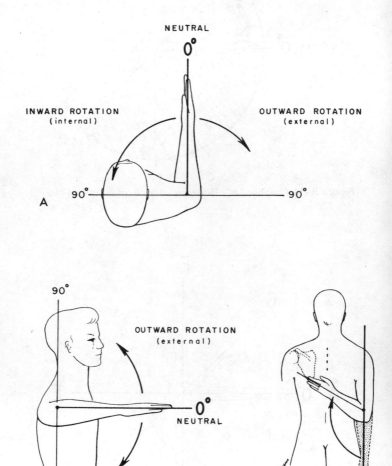

Figure A–13. The shoulder (rotation). *A*, Rotation with arm at side. *B*, Rotation in abduction. *C*, Internal rotation posteriorly.

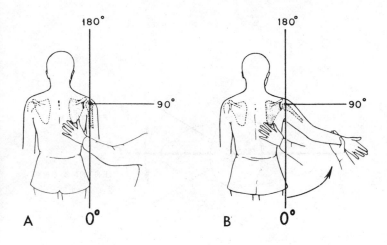

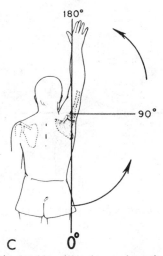

Figure A–14. The shoulder (glenohumeral motion). *A,* Neutral. *B,* Range of true glenohumeral motion. *C,* "Combined" glenohumeral and scapulothoracic motion.

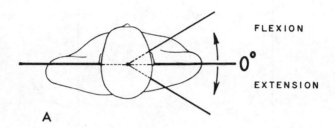

FLEXION

0°

EXTENSION

A

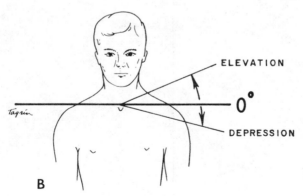

ELEVATION

0°

DEPRESSION

B

Figure A–15. Motion of the shoulder girdle.

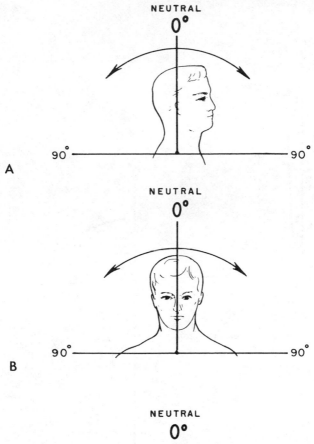

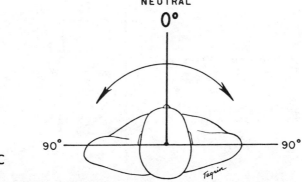

Figure A–16. The cervical spine. *A,* Flexion and extension. *B,* Lateral bend. *C,* Rotation.

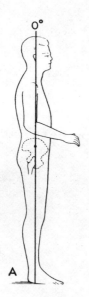

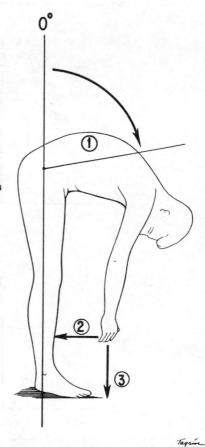

0°

A

① DEGREES OF INCLINATION
OF TRUNK.
(note reversal of
lumbar curve)

② LEVEL OF FINGERTIPS
TO LEG

③ DISTANCE BETWEEN
FINGERTIPS AND FLOOR

B

Figure A–17. The thoracic and lumbar spine (flexion). *A*, Zero starting position. *B*, Methods of measuring flexion.

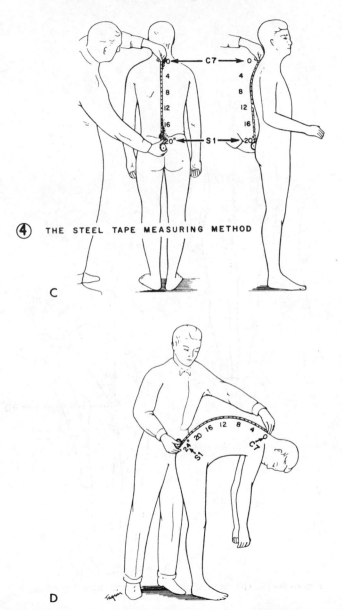

④ THE STEEL TAPE MEASURING METHOD

C

D

Figure A–17 *Continued.* Methods of measuring spinal flexion. *C,* The patient standing erect. *D,* The patient bending forward. (Note the 4 inches in motion [20 in. – 24 in.].)

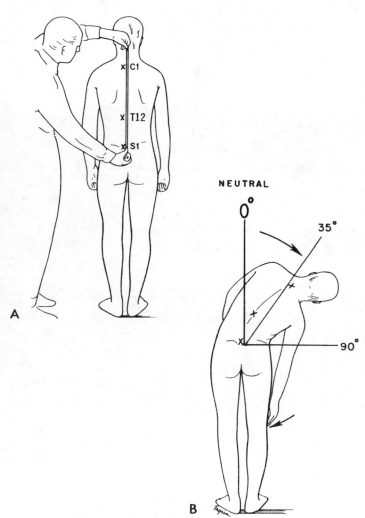

Figure A–18. The thoracic and lumbar spine: lateral bending.

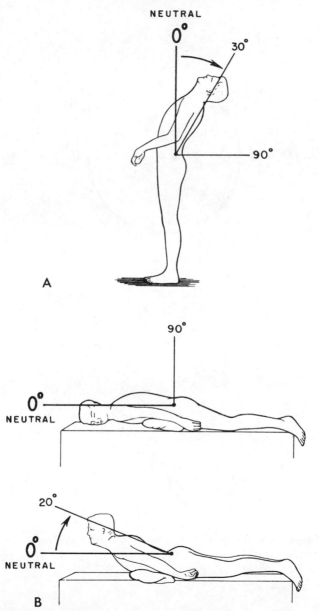

Figure A-19. The thoracic and lumbar spine (extension). *A*, Standing. *B*, Lying prone.

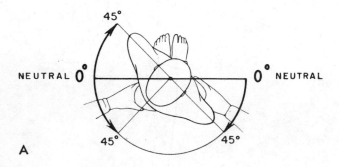

A

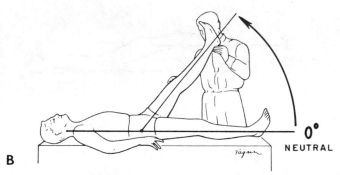

B

Figure A–20. The spine. *A,* Rotation. *B,* Straight leg raising test (passive motion).

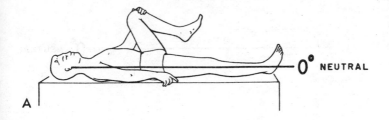

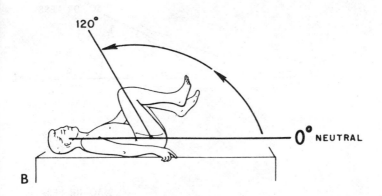

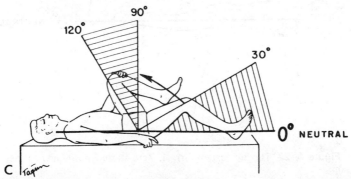

Figure A–21. The hip (flexion). *A*, Zero starting position. *B*, Flexion. *C*, Limited motion in flexion.

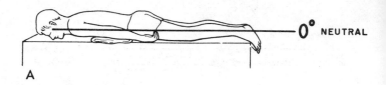

0° NEUTRAL

A

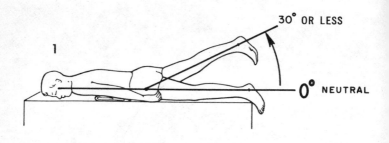

1

30° OR LESS

0° NEUTRAL

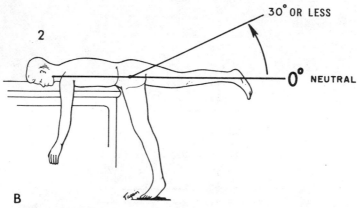

2

30° OR LESS

0° NEUTRAL

B

Figure A–22. The hip (extension). *A,* Zero starting position. *B,* Extension.

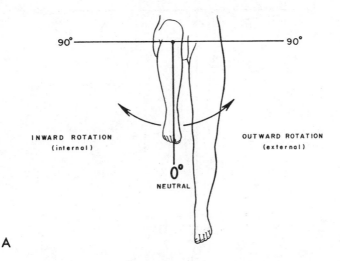

Figure A–23. The hip (rotation). *A*, Rotation in flexion. *B*, Rotation in extension.

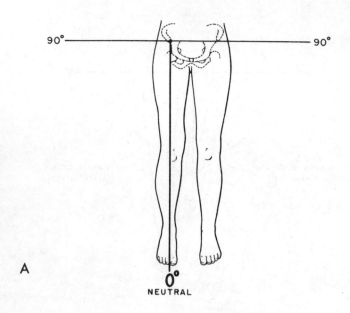

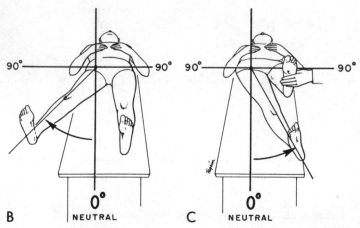

Figure A–24. The hip (abduction and adduction). *A*, Zero starting position. *B*, Abduction. *C*, Adduction.

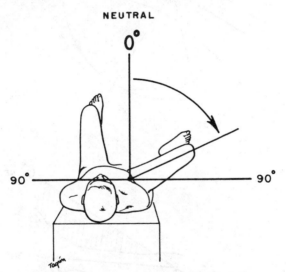

Figure A–25. The hip: abduction in flexion.

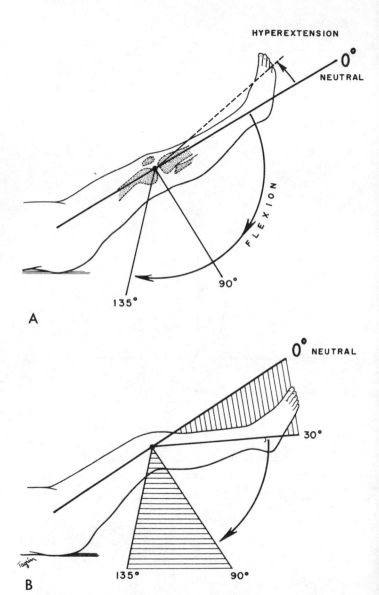

Figure A–26. The knee. *A*, Flexion and hyperextension. *B*, Measurement of limited motion.

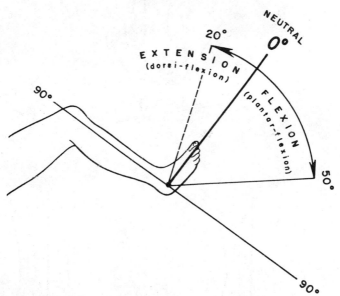

Figure A–27. The ankle: flexion and extension.

HIND PART of the FOOT
(PASSIVE MOTION)

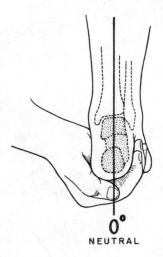

A

0°

NEUTRAL

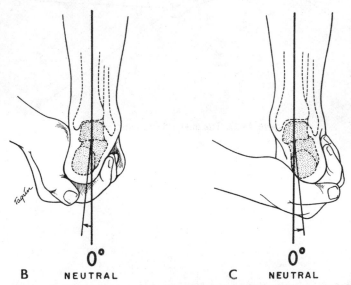

B NEUTRAL   C NEUTRAL

0°   0°

Figure A–28. Hind part of the foot (passive motion). *A*, Zero starting position. *B*, Inversion. *C*, Eversion.

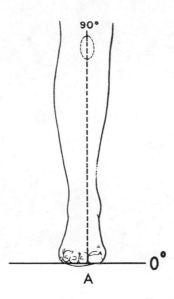

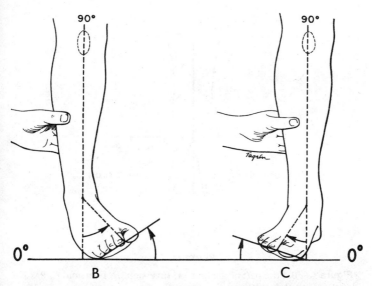

Figure A–29. Fore part of the foot. *A,* Zero starting position. *B,* Inversion (supination, adduction, and plantar flexion). *C,* Eversion (pronation, abduction and dorsiflexion).

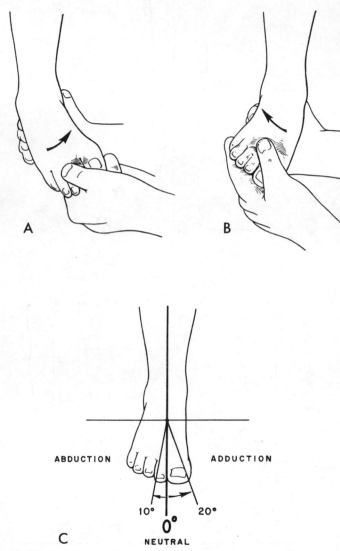

ABDUCTION

ADDUCTION

10° 20°

0°
NEUTRAL

A

B

C

Figure A–30. Fore part of the foot. *A*, Inversion. *B*, Eversion. *C*, Passive adduction and abduction.

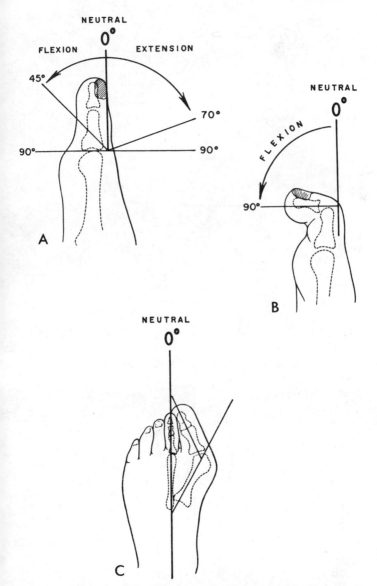

Figure A–31. The great toe. *A*, Metatarsophalangeal joint. *B*, Inter-phalangeal joint. *C*, Hallux valgus.

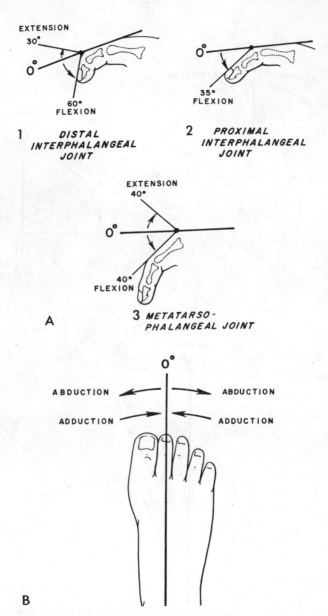

EXTENSION
30°
0°
60°
FLEXION

1 DISTAL
INTERPHALANGEAL
JOINT

0°
35°
FLEXION

2 PROXIMAL
INTERPHALANGEAL
JOINT

EXTENSION
40°
0°
40°
FLEXION

3 METATARSO-
PHALANGEAL JOINT

A

0°

ABDUCTION ← → ABDUCTION
ADDUCTION → ← ADDUCTION

B

Figure A–32. The toes. *A,* Second to fifth toes. *B,* Abduction and adduction (toe spread).

AVERAGE RANGES OF JOINT MOTION

| | SOURCES* | | | | |
JOINT	(1)	(2)	(3)	(4)	AVERAGES
ELBOW =					
FLEXION	150	135	150	150	146
HYPEREXTENSION	0	0	0	0	0
FOREARM =					
PRONATION	80	75	50	80	71
SUPINATION	80	85	90	80	84
WRIST =					
EXTENSION	60	65	90	70	71
FLEXION	70	70		80	73
ULNAR DEV.	30	40	30	30	33
RADIAL DEV.	20	20	15	20	19
THUMB =					
ABDUCTION		55	50	70	58
FLEXION					
I-P Jt.	80	75	90	80	81
M — P	60	50	50	50	53
M — C				15	15
EXTENSION					
Distal Jt.		20	10	20	17
M — P		5	10	0	8
M — C				20	20
FINGERS =					
FLEXION					
Distal Jt.	70	70	90	90	80
Middle Jt.	100	100		100	100
Proximal Jt.	90	90		90	90

AVERAGE RANGES OF JOINT MOTION

SOURCES *

JOINT	(1)	(2)	(3)	(4)	AVERAGES
FINGERS =					
EXTENSION					
Distal Jt.				0	0
Middle Jt.				0	0
Proximal Jt.			45	45	45
SHOULDER =					
FORWARD FLEXION	150	170	130	180	158
HORIZONTAL FLEXION				135	135
BACKWARD EXTENSION	40	30	80	60	53
ABDUCTION	150	170	180	180	170
ADDUCTION	30		45	75	50
ROTATION					
Arm at Side					
Int. Rot.	40	60	90	80	68
Ext. Rot.	90	80	40	60	68
Arm in Abduction (90°)					
Int. Rot.				70	70
Ext. Rot.				90	90
HIP =					
FLEXION	100	110	120	120	113
EXTENSION	30	30	20	30	28
ABDUCTION	40	50	55	45	48
ADDUCTION	20	30	45	30	31
ROTATION					
In Flexion =					
Int. Rot.				45	45
Ext. Rot.				45	45
In Extension =					
Int. Rot.	40	35	20	45	35
Ext. Rot.	50	50	45	45	48
ABDUCTION					
In 90° of flexion			45 to 60		
			(depending on age)		

AVERAGE RANGES OF JOINT MOTION
SOURCES*

JOINT	(1)	(2)	(3)	(4)	AVERAGES
KNEE =					
FLEXION	120	135	145	135	134
HYPEREXTENSION			10	10	10
ANKLE =					
FLEXION (plantar flexion)	40	50	50	50	48
EXTENSION (dorsiflexion)	20	15	15	20	18
HIND FOOT (subtalar) =					
INVERSION				5	5
EVERSION				5	5
FORE FOOT =					
INVERSION	30	35		35	33
EVERSION	20	20		15	18
TOES =					
GREAT TOE					
I-P Jt.					
Flexion	30			90	60
Extension	0			0	0
Proximal Jt.					
Flexion	30	35		45	37
Extension	50	70		70	63
2nd TO 5th TOES =					
FLEXION					
Distal Jt.	50			60	55
Middle Jt.	40			35	38
Proximal Jt.	30			40	35
Extension	40			40	40

AVERAGE RANGES OF JOINT MOTION

SOURCES*

JOINT	(1)	(2)	(3)	(4)	AVERAGES

SPINE =

CERVICAL

FLEXION	30			45	38
EXTENSION	30			45	38
LAT. BENDING	40			45	43
ROTATION	30			60	45

THORACIC AND LUMBAR

FLEXION	90			$\begin{cases} 80 \\ 4'' \end{cases}$	$\begin{cases} 85 \\ 4'' \end{cases}$
EXTENSION	30			20-30	30
LAT. BENDING	20			35	28
ROTATION	30			45	38

*Column (1): From the Journal of the American Medical Association: A Guide to the Evaluation of Permanent Impairment of the Extremities and Back. Special Edition, pp 1–112, Feb 15, 1958.
Column (2): From the Committee of the California Medical Association and the Industrial Accident Commission of the State of California: Evaluation of Industrial Disability. Oxford University Press, 1960.
Column (3): From Clark WA: A system of joint measurements. J Orthop Surg 2:Dec 1920.
Column (4): The Committee on Joint Motion, American Academy of Orthopaedic Surgeons.

3

DERMATOMES

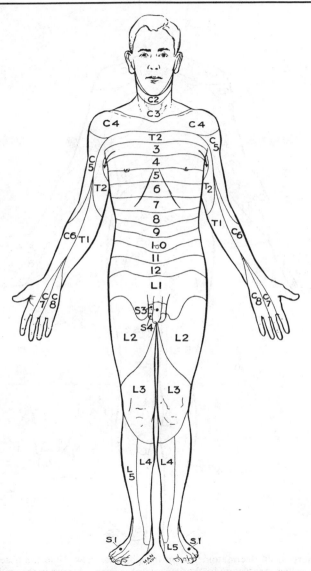

Figure A–33. Segmental innervation of the skin from the anterior aspect. The uppermost dermatome adjoins the cutaneous field of the mandibular division of the trigeminal nerve. The arrows indicate the lateral extensions of dermatome T3. (After Foerster, 1933; from Haymaker W, Woodhall B: Peripheral Nerve Injuries, 2nd ed. Philadelphia, Saunders, 1953.)

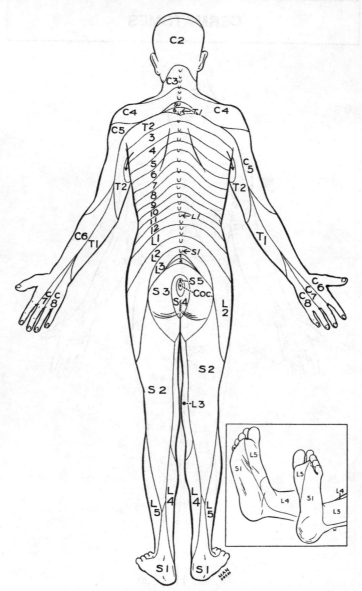

Figure A–34. Dermatomes from the posterior view. Note the absence of cutaneous innervation by the 1st cervical segment. Arrows in the axillary regions indicate the lateral extent of dermatome T3; those in the region of the vertebral column point to the 1st thoracic, 1st lumbar, and 1st sacral spinous processes. (After Foerster, 1933; from Haymaker W, Woodhall B: Peripheral Nerve Injuries, 2nd ed. Philadelphia, Saunders, 1953.)

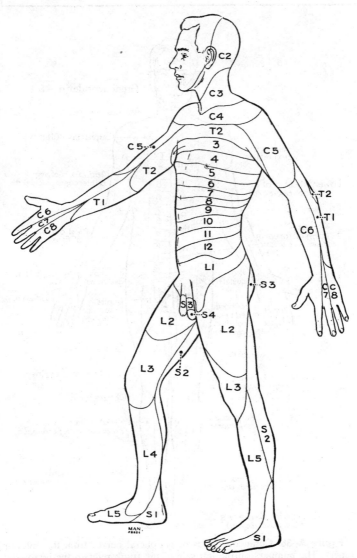

Figure A–35. A side view of the dermatomes. (After Foerster, 1933; from Haymaker W, Woodhall B: Peripheral Nerve Injuries, 2nd ed. Philadelphia, Saunders, 1953.)

4

CUTANEOUS FIELDS

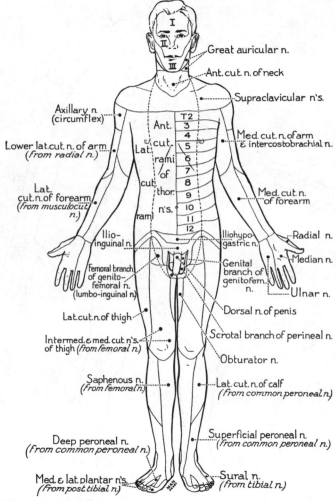

Figure A–36. Cutaneous fields of peripheral nerves from the anterior aspect. The numbers on the left side of the trunk refer to the intercostal nerves. On the right side are shown the cutaneous fields of the lateral and medial branches of the anterior primary rami. The asterisk just beneath the scrotum is in the field of the posterior cutaneous nerve of the thigh. (From Haymaker W, Woodhall B: Peripheral Nerve Injuries, 2nd ed. Philadelphia, Saunders, 1953.)

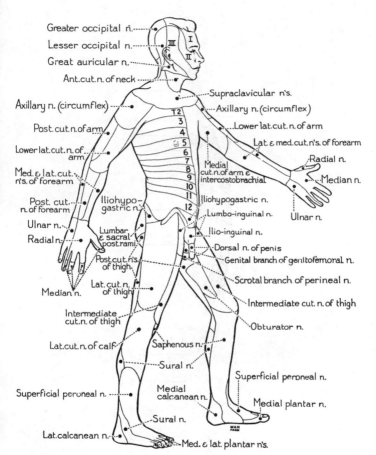

Figure A–37. Side view of the cutaneous fields of peripheral nerves. The face and anterior half of the head are innervated by the three divisions of the trigeminal: I, ophthalmic; II, maxillary; III, mandibular. The fields of the intercostal nerves are indicated by numerals. The unlabeled cutaneous field between the great and 2nd toes is supplied by the deep peroneal nerve. (From Haymaker W, Woodhall B: Peripheral Nerve Injuries, 2nd ed. Philadelphia, Saunders, 1953.)

ALIGNMENT OF SPINAL SEGMENTS WITH VERTEBRAE

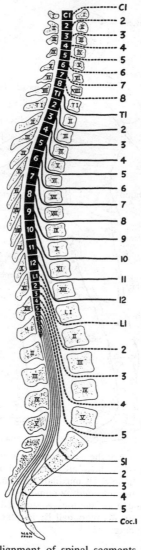

Figure A–38. The alignment of spinal segments with vertebrae. The bodies and spinous processes of the vertebrae are indicated by Roman numerals. (From Haymaker W, Woodhall B: Peripheral Nerve Injuries, 2nd ed. Philadelphia, Saunders, 1953.)

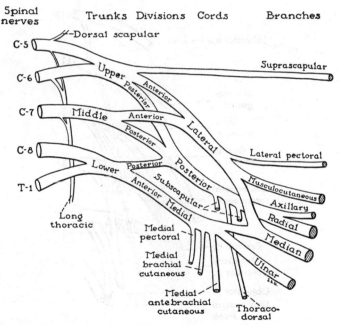

Figure A–39. A diagram of the brachial plexus. The small nerve to the subclavius, from the upper trunk, is omitted. (Reproduced, with permission, from Hollinshead WH, Jenkins DB: Functional Anatomy of the Limbs and Back, 5th ed. Philadelphia, Saunders, 1981.)

7

LUMBAR PLEXUS

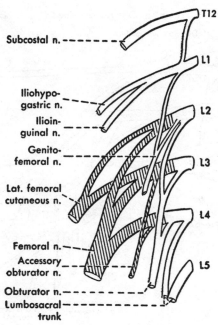

Figure A–40. A diagram of the lumbar plexus. The posterior portions of the plexus are shaded. (Reproduced, with permission, from Hollinshead WH, Jenkins DB: Functional Anatomy of the Limbs and Back, 5th ed. Philadelphia, Saunders, 1981.)

SACRAL PLEXUS

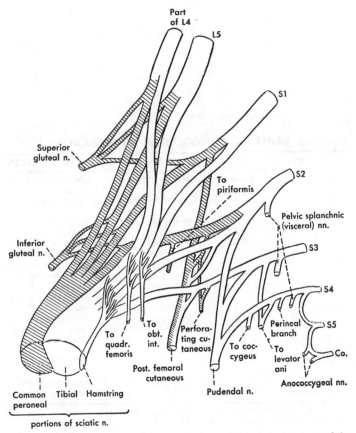

Figure A–41. A diagram of the sacral plexus. The posterior parts of the plexus are shaded. (Reproduced, with permission, from Hollinshead WH, Jenkins DB: Functional Anatomy of the Limbs and Back, 5th ed. Philadelphia, Saunders, 1981.)

MUSCLES, PERIPHERAL NERVES, SPINAL ROOTS

NERVES AND MUSCLES OF THE SHOULDER*

NERVE	ORIGIN	MUSCLE	CHIEF ACTION
Accessory	Cranial	Sternocleidomastoid	Lateral flex and rotate head
Nn. to levator scapulae	C3, 4	Levator scapulae	Elevate shoulder tip
Dorsal scapular	C5	Both rhomboidei	Retract scapula
N. to subclavius	C5, 6	Subclavius	Depress clavicle
Axillary	C5, 6	Teres minor	Externally rotate and abduct arm
Upper subscapular	C5, 6	Subscapularis	Internally rotate arm
Lower subscapular	C5, 6	Subscapularis	Internally rotate arm
		Teres major	Externally and internally rotate arm
Suprascapular	C5, 6	Supraspinatus	Abduct arm
		Infraspinatus	Externally rotate arm
Long thoracic	C5, 6, 7	Serratus anterior	Upward rotate arm
Lateral pectoral	C5, 6, 7	Upper pectoralis major	Adduct-flex arm
Medial pectoral	C8, T1	Lower pectoralis major	Adduct-extend arm
		Pectoralis minor	Depress shoulder
Thoracodorsal	C6, 7, 8	Latissimus dorsi	Extend-adduct arm

*Adapted from Hollinshead WH, Jenkins DB: Functional Anatomy of the Limbs and Back, 5th ed. Philadelphia, Saunders, 1981.

NERVES AND MUSCLES OF THE ARM*

NERVE AND ORIGIN	MUSCLE	SEGMENTAL INNER- VATION	CHIEF ACTION
Musculocutaneous	Biceps	C5, 6	Flex-supinate forearm
C5–C7	Coracobrachialis	C5, 6, 7	Adduct-flex forearm
	Brachialis	C5, 6	Flex forearm
Radial	Triceps	C5, 6, 7, 8	Extend forearm
C5–C8	Anconeus	C6, 7	Extend forearm

THE FLEXOR FOREARM

NERVE AND ORIGIN	MUSCLE	SEGMENTAL INNER- VATION	CHIEF ACTION
Median	Pronator teres	C6, 7	Pronate forearm
C5–T1	Pronator quadratus	C7–T1	Pronate forearm
	Flexor carpi radialis	C6, 7	Flex wrist
	Palmaris longus	C7, 8	Flex wrist
	Flexor digitorum superficialis	C7–T1	Flex middle phalanges
	Flexor pollicis longus	C7–T1	Flex distal thumb phalanges
	Flexor digitorum profundus, radial part	C8, T1	Flex distal phalanges of digits II, III
Ulnar	Flexor digitorum profundus, ulnar part	C8, T1	Flex distal phalanges of digits IV, V
C8, T1	Flexor carpi ulnaris	C8, T1	Flex-adduct wrist

*Adapted from Hollinshead WH, Jenkins DB: Functional Anatomy of the Limbs and Back, 5th ed. Philadelphia, Saunders, 1981.

NERVES AND MUSCLES OF THE EXTENSOR FOREARM*

NERVE AND ORIGIN	MUSCLE	SEGMENTAL INNER- VATION	CHIEF ACTION
Radial C5, 6, 7, 8	Brachioradialis	C5, 6	Flex elbow
	Extensor carpi radialis longus and brevis	C6, 7	Extend-abduct wrist
	Extensor carpi ulnaris	C6, 7, 8	Extend-adduct wrist
	Supinator	C5, 6	Supinate forearm
	Extensor digitorum	C6, 7, 8	Extend all joints of digits II–V
	Extensor digiti minimi	C6, 7, 8	Extend all joints of digit V
	Extensor indicis	C7, 8	Extend all joints of digit II
	Extensor pollicis longus	C7, 8	Extend both phalanges; extend, adduct metacarpal of thumb
	Extensor pollicis brevis	C6, 7	Extend proximal phalanx and metacarpal of thumb; abduct wrist
	Abductor pollicis longus	C6, 7	Extend, abduct thumb; flex, abduct wrist

*Adapted from Hollinshead WH, Jenkins DB: Functional Anatomy of the Limbs and Back, 5th ed. Philadelphia, Saunders, 1981.

NERVES AND MUSCLES OF THE HAND*

NERVE AND ORIGIN	MUSCLE	CHIEF ACTION
Median C5–T1	Abductor pollicis brevis	Abduct thumb
	Flexor pollicis brevis, superficial head	Flex MCP joint of thumb
	Opponens pollicis	Oppose thumb
	Lumbricals I, II	Extend IP joints; flex MCP joints of digits II, III
Ulnar C8, T1	Flexor pollicis brevis, deep head	Flex MCP joint of thumb
	Adductor pollicis	Adduct metacarpal, flex MCP joint of thumb
	Abductor digiti minimi	Abduct digit V
	Flexor digiti minimi brevis	Flex MCP joint of digit V
	Opponens digiti minimi	Cup hand
	Lumbricals III, IV	Extend IP joints; flex MCP joints of digits IV, V
	Palmar interossei	Adduct digits II, IV, V; flex MCP and extend IP joints
	Dorsal interossei	Abduct digits II, III, IV; flex MCP and extend IP joints

*Adapted from Hollinshead WH, Jenkins DB: Functional Anatomy of the Limbs and Back, 5th ed. Philadelphia, Saunders, 1981.
Notes: MCP = metacarpophalangeal.
      IP = interphalangeal.

NERVES AND MUSCLES OF THE THIGH*

NERVE AND ORIGIN	MUSCLE	SEGMENTAL INNER-VATION	CHIEF ACTION
L2, 3, 4	Iliopsoas	L2, 3, 4	Flex hip
Femoral L2, 3, 4	Sartorius	L2, 3	Flex, rotate hip and knee
	Quadriceps	L2, 3, 4	Extend knee
	Pectineus	L2, 3	Flex, adduct hip
Obturator	Pectineus (sometimes)	L2, 3	Flex, adduct hip
L2, 3, 4	Adductor longus	L2, 3	Adduct, flex hip
	Adductor brevis	L3, 4	Adduct, flex hip
	Gracilis	L3, 4	Adduct hip; flex knee
	Adductor magnus (ant. part)	L3, 4	Adduct, flex hip
	Obturator externus	L3, 4	Externally rotate hip

*Adapted from Hollinshead WH, Jenkins DB: Functional Anatomy of the Limbs and Back, 5th ed. Philadelphia, Saunders, 1981.

NERVES AND MUSCLES OF THE BUTTOCK AND POSTERIOR THIGH*

NERVE AND ORIGIN	MUSCLE	SEGMENTAL INNER-VATION	CHIEF ACTION
Superior gluteal	Gluteus medius	L4–S1	Abduct-externally rotate hip
L4–S1	Gluteus minimus	L4–S1	Abduct-internally rotate hip
	Tensor fasciae latae	L4–S1	Flex-internally rotate hip
Inferior gluteal L5–S2	Gluteus maximus	L5–S2	Extend-adduct hip
N. to piriformis S1, 2	Piriformis	S1, 2	Externally rotate hip
N. to obturator internus and	Obturator internus	L5–S2	Externally rotate hip
superior gemellus L5–S2	Superior gemellus	L5–S2	Externally rotate hip
N. to quadratus femoris and	Inferior gemellus	L4–S1	Externally rotate hip
inferior gemellus L4–S1	Quadratus femoris	L4–S1	Externally rotate hip
Tibial	Semitendinosus	L5, S1	Extend hip, flex knee
L4–S3	Semimembranosus	L5, S1	Extend hip, flex knee
	Biceps, long head	L5–S2	Extend hip, flex knee
	Adductor magnus, posterior part	L4, 5	Extend hip
Common peroneal L4–S2	Biceps, short head	L5, S1	Flex knee

*Adapted from Hollinshead WH, Jenkins DB: Functional Anatomy of the Limbs and Back, 5th ed. Philadelphia, Saunders, 1981.

NERVES AND MUSCLES OF THE LEG*

NERVE AND ORIGIN	MUSCLE	SEGMENTAL INNER-VATION	CHIEF ACTION
Tibial	Gastrocnemius	S1, 2	Plantar flex ankle
L4–S3	Soleus	S1, 2	Plantar flex ankle
	Plantaris	L4–S1	Plantar flex ankle
	Popliteus	L5, S1	Rotate, flex knee
	Tibialis posterior	L5, S1	Adduct, invert foot
	Flexor digitorum longus	L5, S1	Flex four lateral toes
	Flexor hallucis longus	L5–S2	Flex big toe
Superficial peroneal L4–S1	Peroneus longus	L4–S1	Evert foot
	Peroneus brevis	L4–S1	Evert foot
Deep peroneal	Tibialis anterior	L4–S1	Invert, dorsiflex foot
L4–S2	Extensor digitorum longus	L4–S1	Extend four lateral toes and dorsiflex foot
	Peroneus tertius	L4–S1	Evert, dorsiflex foot
	Extensor hallucis longus	L4–S1	Extend big toe

*Adapted from Hollinshead WH, Jenkins DB: Functional Anatomy of the Limbs and Back, 5th ed. Philadelphia, Saunders, 1981.

NERVES AND MUSCLES OF THE FOOT*

NERVE AND ORIGIN	MUSCLE	SEGMENTAL INNER-VATION	CHIEF ACTION
Medial plantar L5, S1	Abductor hallucis	L5, S1	Abduct-flex big toe
	Flexor hallucis brevis	L5, S1	Flex big toe
	Flexor digitorum brevis	L5, S1	Flex four lateral toes
	First lumbrical	L5, S1	Flex toe II
Lateral plantar	Three lateral lumbricals	S1, 2	Flex three lateral toes
S1, 2	Flexor digiti minimi brevis	S1, 2	Flex toe V
	Abductor digiti minimi	S1, 2	Abduct toe V
	Adductor hallucis	S1, 2	Adduct big toe
	Plantar interossei	S1, 2	Adduct, flex three lateral toes
	Dorsal interossei	S1, 2	Abduct, flex toes II, III, IV
Deep peroneal L4–S2	Extensor digitorum and hallucis brevis	L5, S1	Extend toes

*Adapted from Hollinshead WH, Jenkins DB: Functional Anatomy of the Limbs and Back, 5th ed. Philadelphia, Saunders, 1981.

DISTRIBUTION OF MAJOR PERIPHERAL NERVES

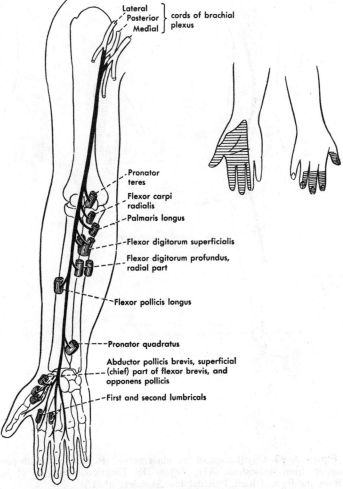

Figure A–42. Distribution of the median nerve. (Reproduced, with permission, from Hollinshead WH, Jenkins DB: Functional Anatomy of the Limbs and Back, 5th ed. Philadelphia, Saunders, 1981.)

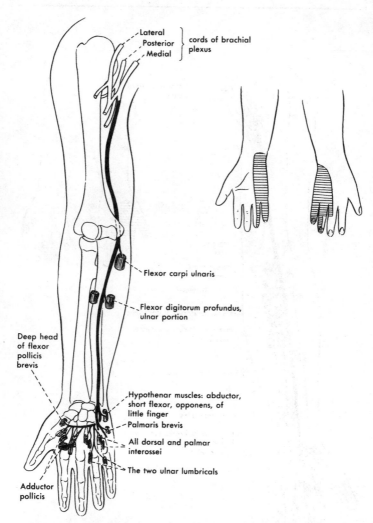

Figure A–43. Distribution of the ulnar nerve. (Reproduced, with permission, from Hollinshead WH, Jenkins DB: Functional Anatomy of the Limbs and Back, 5th ed. Philadelphia, Saunders, 1981.)

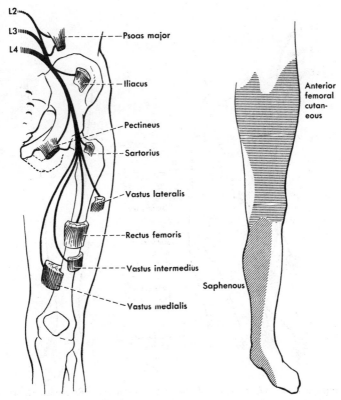

Figure A–44. Distribution of the femoral nerve. (Reproduced, with permission, from Hollinshead WH, Jenkins DB: Functional Anatomy of the Limbs and Back, 5th ed. Philadelphia, Saunders, 1981.)

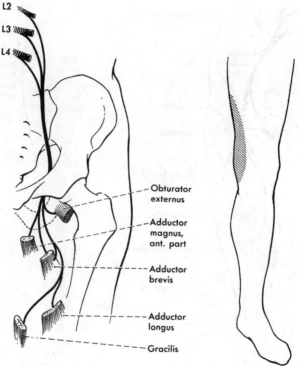

L2

L3

L4

Obturator
externus

Adductor
magnus,
ant. part

Adductor
brevis

Adductor
longus

Gracilis

Figure A–45. Distribution of the obturator nerve. (Reproduced, with permission, from Hollinshead WH, Jenkins DB: Functional Anatomy of the Limbs and Back, 5th ed. Philadelphia, Saunders, 1981.)

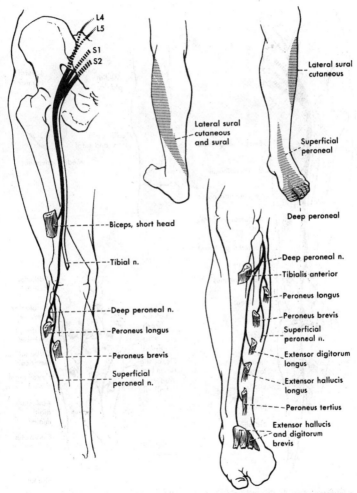

Figure A–46. Distribution of the common peroneal nerve. (Reproduced, with permission, from Hollinshead WH, Jenkins DB: Functional Anatomy of the Limbs and Back, 5th ed. Philadelphia, Saunders, 1981.)

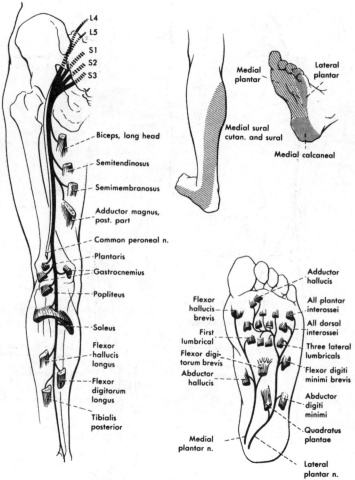

Figure A–47. Distribution of the tibial nerve. (Reproduced, with permission, from Hollinshead WH, Jenkins DB: Functional Anatomy of the Limbs and Back, 5th ed. Philadelphia, Saunders, 1981.)

Note: Numbers in *italics* refer to illustrations; numbers followed by (t) refer to tables.